Pharmacology

CASE STUDY WORKBOOK

Kathy A. Putman, RN, MSN

Nursing Faculty
Saginaw Valley State University
Crystal M. Lange College of Health and Human Services
University Center, Michigan

JONES AND BARTLETT PUBLISHERS

Sudbury, Massachusetts

BOSTON   TORONTO   LONDON   SINGAPORE

World Headquarters

Jones and Bartlett Publishers
40 Tall Pine Drive
Sudbury, MA 01776
978-443-5000
info@jbpub.com
www.jbpub.com

Jones and Bartlett Publishers
Canada
6339 Ormindale Way
Mississauga, Ontario L5V 1J2
Canada

Jones and Bartlett Publishers
International
Barb House, Barb Mews
London W6 7PA
United Kingdom

Jones and Bartlett's books and products are available through most bookstores and online booksellers. To contact Jones and Bartlett Publishers directly, call 800-832-0034, fax 978-443-8000, or visit our website, www.jbpub.com.

Substantial discounts on bulk quantities of Jones and Bartlett's publications are available to corporations, professional associations, and other qualified organizations. For details and specific discount information, contact the special sales department at Jones and Bartlett via the above contact information or send an email to specialsales@jbpub.com.

The author, editor, and publisher have made every effort to provide accurate information. However, they are not responsible for errors, omissions, or for any outcomes related to the use of the contents of this book and take no responsibility for the use of the products and procedures described. Treatments and side effects described in this book may not be applicable to all people; likewise, some people may require a dose or experience a side effect that is not described herein. Drugs and medical devices are discussed that may have limited availability controlled by the Food and Drug Administration (FDA) for use only in a research study or clinical trial. Research, clinical practice, and government regulations often change the accepted standard in this field. When consideration is being given to use of any drug in the clinical setting, the health care provider or reader is responsible for determining FDA status of the drug, reading the package insert, and reviewing prescribing information for the most up-to-date recommendations on dose, precautions, and contraindications, and determining the appropriate usage for the product. This is especially important in the case of drugs that are new or seldom used.

Production Credits
Publisher: Kevin Sullivan
Acquisitions Editor: Amy Sibley
Associate Editor: Patricia Donnelly
Editorial Assistant: Rachel Shuster
Associate Production Editor: Lisa Cerrone
Marketing Manager: Rebecca Wasley
V.P., Manufacturing and Inventory Control: Therese Connell
Composition: Graphic World
Cover Design: Scott Moden
Cover Image: © drKaczmar/ShutterStock, Inc.
Printing and Binding: Courier Stoughton
Cover Printing: Courier Stoughton

Library of Congress Cataloging-in-Publication Data
Putman, Kathy A.
  Pharmacology case study workbook / Kathy A. Putman.
    p. ; cm.
  Includes bibliographical references and index.
  ISBN 978-0-7637-7613-8 (pbk.)
  1. Clinical pharmacology—Case studies. 2. Chemotherapy—Case studies. I. Title.
  [DNLM: 1. Nursing Assessment—methods—Case Reports. 2. Drug Therapy—nursing—Case
Reports. 3. Pharmacology, Clinical—methods—Case Reports. WY 100.4 P988p 2011]
  RM301.28P88 2011
  615'.1—dc22

                                                                              2010000713

6048

Printed in the United States of America
14 13 12 11 10   10 9 8 7 6 5 4 3 2 1

Table of Contents

Preface

Pharmacology Case Study Workbook was developed after years of teaching different levels of nursing students. In it you will find numerous real-life situations and patients for discussion; however, this workbook is much more than a collection of diseases and the medications that go with them. We as healthcare providers are aware that no patient comes with just one medical diagnosis. Oftentimes, one healthcare issue can, and usually does, lead to another. It takes time for students to see the bigger picture, and at the beginning, most students attempt to compartmentalize diseases and medications.

Not only have I taught different levels of nursing students, but I have also facilitated learning in different states and settings, both in and out of the hospital. Students have spanned the continuum from level one in fundamentals to senior students in a Level I trauma center. Whatever their level, students have learned that medications are a large part of patient care and medication errors are always possible. I wanted students to understand medication reconciliations, the consequences of medication errors, and safety with regard to medication administration. I also wanted students to be aware that medications sometimes interact with each other, producing unintended or detrimental consequences in the patient. I researched different resources, but I could not find what worked best for my students and me. I needed a different approach, so I created my own.

Upon observation, I realized that students reviewed a patient's entire chart (gathered labs and diagnostic tests) and left the patient's medications until last, thinking they were not all that important. They then proceeded to miss the PRN medications or think the "as needed" medications were not really important because they were not given on a regular basis. Additionally, students were compartmentalizing the medications and not seeing the bigger picture.

As a result, I began having students essentially work backward. Instead of the usual procedure in which students reviewed the chart and wrote down the labs and diagnostic tests along with a primary and secondary medical diagnosis, I had students review the medications and write up a synopsis of them. Essentially, students had only the patient's medication record and the medication reconciliation form at the beginning of care. This made some students anxious, mostly because they had to develop questions.

Many students realized that patients were often taking 10 or more medications, which led to discussions about polypharmacy and pharmacokinetics. They noticed if patients had been prescribed a hematopoietic or immune system medication, which led to discussions about which lab values needed to be reviewed or drawn. Students realized that many patients had been prescribed pain medications or were taking over-the-counter pain medications, which led to discussions about the different types and classifications of pain.

As instructors, we want students to develop a diagnosis independent of the medical model diagnosis. By having students develop care as I have described, they can arrive at interventions and outcomes that are independent of the medical diagnosis. This forces students to look at the information without a medical diagnosis to use as a crutch; only after developing a patient's diagnosis are students allowed to review the medical chart.

I have found that this method works for any level of student, and for students who study patients and medications. With no penalty for wrong answers, students had the freedom to think and collaborate. It also allowed me the ability to see where and how their thoughts might be leading them off course. This works well for those who are accustomed to using a Socratic method of teaching, and for teachers who function in a lecture mode in the classroom.

In *Pharmacology Case Study Workbook*, I have gathered and prepared some of the more common cases my students have seen in the different healthcare settings. There are several ways this workbook can be used. It functions as a supplement to a pharmacology textbook, but it can also be used with any drug handbook without a pharmacology text. Additionally, students can use this text individually or as some have done, in a group discussion setting. If this text works for you as it has for me, it will have your students thinking and asking questions.

The questions found in this workbook are straightforward; however, they require that the student look at the big picture and not compartmentalize the medications or the patient. The student has to assimilate the information presented and acquired knowledge to come up with answers. The workbook includes vocabulary related to each case, guided inquiries to move the students along in the study of the patient and the medications, and physical assessment findings. Cases conclude with a synopsis of what happened to the patient.

Within the cases you will discover several questions and answers that students and I have discussed. However, I have left some of the questions unanswered deliberately. This is to give the instructor the ability to question students on a given topic, issue, or subject; to model Socratic questioning for students; or to help students analyze a concept or line of reasoning. Students should learn the discipline of Socratic questioning so that they can begin to use it when analyzing multifaceted issues. These types of issues are found often, particularly in health care. By understanding and assessing the thinking of others and themselves and in following the implications, students are more likely to see different conclusions. This method teaches students to dig beneath the surface of any idea, and teaches both students and teachers the value of developing questioning minds in cultivating deep learning. I also encourage students to question my answers and ask me to explain them. I do not expect them to do something I am not willing to do myself.

Some of my colleagues may think that this workbook is beyond the scope of nursing and should be left to the physician; however, I disagree. Those who work in a clinical setting are aware of the need to work as an interprofessional colleague. Students of medicine, pharmacy, and nursing (practical, associate, or baccalaureate) and their instructors will find this workbook to be helpful. Any material that helps a student of any profession to work more safely and teaches us to speak the same language in collaboration leads to better health care. This material has worked for me and my students. Hopefully, you will find it useful as well.

Be encouraged,
Kathy A. Putman, RN, MSN

Abbreviations

ACE	angiotensin-converting enzyme
ANA	antinuclear antibody
ANC	absolute neutrophil count
AV	arteriovenous
BNP	B-type natriuretic peptide
BPH	benign prostate hypertrophy
BUN	blood urea nitrogen
CAD	coronary artery disease
C&S	culture and sensitivity
CBC	complete blood count
CCB	calcium channel blocker
CINV	chemotherapy-induced nausea and vomiting
CK	creatinine kinase
COPD	chronic obstructive pulmonary disease
CRP	C-reactive protein
CT	computed tomography
CTZ	chemoreceptor trigger zone
CXR	chest X-ray
DIC	disseminated intravascular coagulation
DM	diabetes mellitus
DMARD	disease-modifying antirheumatic
DNR	do not resuscitate
DRE	digital rectal exam
DVT	deep vein thrombosis
ECG	electrocardiogram
EMG	electromyography
ESR	erythrocyte sedimentation rate
ESRF	end-stage renal failure
FBS	fasting blood sugar
FDA	Food and Drug Administration
Fe	iron
FUO	fever of unknown origin
GERD	gastroesophageal reflux disease
GFR	glomerular filtration rate
GI	gastrointestinal
HDL	high-density lipoprotein

ICU	intensive care unit
IM	intramuscular
INR	international normalized ratio
IU	international units
IV	intravenous(ly)
JVD	jugular vein distention
KUB	kidney, ureter, bladder
LDL	low-density lipoprotein
MRSA	methicillin-resistant *Staphylococcus aureus*
MMSE	mini-mental state exam
MRI	magnetic resonance imaging
MS	multiple sclerosis
MTX	methotrexate
MVI	multiple vitamins for infusion
NANDA	North American Nursing Diagnosis Association
NGT	nasogastric tube
NIC	Nursing Interventions Classification
NOC	Nursing Outcomes Classification
NS	normal saline
NSAID	nonsteroidal anti-inflammatory drug
NYHA	New York Heart Association
OA	osteoarthritis
OTC	over the counter
PA	pulmonary artery
PB	phenobarbital
PD	Parkinson's disease
PEG	percutaneous endoscopic gastrostomy
PET	positron emission tomography
PICC	peripherally inserted central catheter
PM	polymyositis
PACU	postanesthesia care unit
PSA	prostate-specific antigen
PT	prothrombin time
RA	rheumatoid arthritis
RBC	red blood cell
RAAS	renin-angiotensin-aldosterone system
SARS	severe acute respiratory syndrome
SBAR	situation, background, assessment, recommendation
SGOT	serum glutamic oxaloacetic transaminase
SGPT	serum glutamic pyruvic transaminase
SSRI	selective serotonin reuptake inhibitor

T.	temperature
TEE	transesophageal echocardiogram
T_4	thyroxine
TIA	transient ischemic attack
TPN	total parenteral nutrition
T_3	triiodothyronine
UC	ulcerative colitis
UTI	urinary tract infection
WBC	white blood cell

Case Study Inquiry

1

Vocabulary

🔑 Self-Query

Before attempting to work the case study, define each of the vocabulary words. Although the words may have several subheadings, it will give you a place to begin your inquiry.

Beriberi (dry, wet, cerebral)

_____

Chronic alcoholism

_____

Chronic illness

_____

Cirrhosis of the liver

_____

Depression

_____

Gastrointestinal (GI) bleed

_____

Hypertension

_____

Left-sided heart failure

_____

Lethargy

_____

Medication reconciliation

_____

Over the counter

_____

Transient ischemic attack (TIA)

_____

Wernicke-Korsakoff syndrome

_____

You are attempting to do a medication reconciliation for an individual brought into the emergency department by ambulance. She was discovered lethargic on her kitchen floor by her daughter, who presents you with a list of medications. She wrote them down in a hurry while leaving the house. Unfortunately, she did not think to bring the medication bottles. All you know is that the individual is a 66-year-old white female accompanied by her daughter.

Recent History

Nausea and vomiting over the past few days; diarrhea in the last 24 hours; notable stumbling during ambulation. The daughter stated that she attempted to phone her mother and was unable to understand her responses. When she arrived at her mother's house 20 minutes later, she found her on the floor. The daughter stated, "I feared a heart attack or a stroke, and I called 911."

Home Medications

Aspirin (Ecotrin) 325 mg orally daily

Cefpodoxime (Vantin) 200 mg twice a day orally

Chlordiazepoxide hydrochloride (Librium) 25 mg 3 times a day orally

Furosemide (Lasix) 40 mg every day orally

Lorazepam (Ativan) 1 mg orally, 1–2 every 2–4 hours as needed

Nitro paste 1 inch every 6 hours topically

Oxazepam (Serax) 15 mg orally every 12 hours

Potassium chloride 20 mEq every day orally

Thiamine hydrochloride (B1) 100-mg tab daily

? Self-Query

Using a drug book or pharmacology text that contains the mechanism of action, unlabeled uses, and pharmacokinetics for medications, answer the following questions. Make answers specific to this scenario.

What do I know about these medications? Do I know the recommended dose of, the recommended route for, and the best time of day to give these medications? Do I know what lab results I need regarding each medication? Do I know the approved use of each medication? Do I know the most common diseases treated by the listed medications? Are any off-label uses approved for each drug?

Aspirin

_____

_____

Cefpodoxime

_____

_____

Chlordiazepoxide hydrochloride

_____

_____

Furosemide

_____

_____

Lorazepam

_____

_____

Nitro paste

_____

_____

Oxazepam

_____

_____

Potassium chloride

_____

_____

Thiamine hydrochloride

_____

_____

Do I know the individual's past medical history by looking at the medication list?

_____

_____

Allergies

Meperidine (Demerol)

? Self-Query

Do I know why meperidine is used?

_____

Do I know the signs and symptoms of an adverse reaction to meperidine?

_____

Do I know meperidine's classification?

_____

What is the metabolite of meperidine? What is a major side effect of this metabolite?

_____

Body Systems

? Self-Query

Be prepared to defend your answers.

Can I place each medication under the body system that it commonly affects?

Neurological

_____

Cardiovascular

_____

Hematological

_____

Pulmonary

_____

Gastrointestinal

_____

Nutrition

_____

Genitourinary/renal

_____

Musculoskeletal

_____

Endocrine

_____

Integumentary

_____

Immune

_____

Pain/comfort

_____

Mechanism of Action
❓ Self-Query

Does the individual's medical history have an effect on the pharmacokinetics of each drug?

_____

_____

What contraindications do I need to address regarding the medications and medical history?

_____

_____

Nursing Process
❓ Self-Query

What nursing assessment will I do regarding each medication? What planning and implementation do I need to conduct for each medication? How do I evaluate each medication's effectiveness?

Aspirin

_____

_____

Cefpodoxime

_____

_____

Chlordiazepoxide hydrochloride

_____

_____

Furosemide

_____

_____

Lorazepam

_____

_____

Nitro paste

_____

_____

Oxazepam

_____

_____

Potassium chloride

_____

_____

Thiamine hydrochloride

_____

_____

Do I need to be concerned with geriatric considerations for this individual?

_____

Physical Assessment Findings

Neurological Assessment

Acute confusion and slurred speech; decreased consciousness; memory disturbance when able to answer questions; pupils equal, round, and reactive to light.

Cardiovascular and Hematological Assessment

Enzymes: negative, BNP negative, K+ 3.0, S_1S_2 monitor reveals sinus of 50.
Blood pressure 90/50, no edema, extremities pale, capillary refill at 3 seconds.
Bruising to upper extremities and bruising noted on shins bilaterally.

Pulmonary Assessment

Faint crackles heard throughout, respiratory rate 12 per minute, noted clubbing on 4/L oxygen.

Gastrointestinal Assessment

Hyperactive bowel sounds, poor dentations, diarrhea since admitted to the emergency room.

Genitourinary Assessment

Foley inserted, foul odorous output noted. No blood noted.

Musculoskeletal Assessment

Noted inability to coordinate movements, elevated CRP.

Endocrine Assessment

No exophthalmia, no hirsutism, no slow healing wounds, no goiter.

Integumentary Assessment

Bruising to upper extremities and bruising noted on shins bilaterally. IV site to right antecubital 0.9% NS.

Immune Assessment

No palpable lymph nodes, no inflammation noted in joints.

Pain/Comfort Assessment

Grimace to minimal nail bed pressure.

Physician Orders

0.9% NS at 125 mL/hr

Potassium chloride 40 mEq IV

Flumazenil (Romazicon) 0.2 mg IV

Thiamine 100 mg IV

Ciprofloxacin (Cipro) 400 mg IV every 12 hours

Consult mental heath and transfer to neurological floor

Self-Query

What classification is each medication? Why is each medication usually given? How is each medication usually given? Do I know why the physician ordered each medication for this individual?

Potassium chloride

_____

_____

Flumazenil

_____

_____

Thiamine

_____

_____

Ciprofloxacin

_____

_____

Nursing Process

Self-Query

What nursing assessment will I perform regarding each medication? What planning and implementation do I need to conduct for each medication? How do I evaluate each medication's effectiveness?

Potassium chloride

_____

_____

Flumazenil

_____

_____

Thiamine

_____

_____

Ciprofloxacin

_____

_____

What do I think was the final diagnosis?

_____

Synopsis

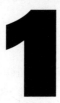

Because you can find answers to the self-queries in numerous texts, you will not find the answers to all of them here. However, you will find discussion of the individual case. The scenario relates to substance abuse; therefore, purposefully look into the medication use and vocabulary as they relate to substance abuse patients.

Vocabulary

When reviewing the vocabulary words, you might want to ask several questions: who, what, where, when, why, and how. This should give you a much broader understanding of each word.

Use the example for medication reconciliation in defining all the vocabulary words. Instead of answering, "The medication reconciliation compares all of a patient's medication orders with all the medications that he or she has been taking," ask:

What are **medication reconciliations**? Who performs medication reconciliations? Where are they done? When are they done? Why are they done? How are they done?

☑ Self-Query: Possible Answers

When defining the remainder of the vocabulary words, you should ask the following questions:

What is the pathophysiology of **beriberi (dry, wet, cerebral)**? Who develops beriberi? What is the treatment? What body system is affected?

What is **chronic alcoholism**? When does a person become an alcoholic?

What is the definition of a **chronic illness**? Who is at risk for a chronic illness?

What is the pathophysiology of **cirrhosis**? Who develops cirrhosis? What is the treatment? What body system is affected?

What are the physical causes of **depression**? Who is at risk for depression? How does chronic illness lead to depression?

What are the medications that can cause gastric bleeds? What medications are used to treat **GI bleeds**?

What commonly causes essential (primary) and secondary **hypertension**? How did essential hypertension obtain its name?

What is the pathophysiology for **left-sided heart failure**? Who is at risk?

Who develops **lethargy**? What causes lethargy?

What defines a drug as **over the counter**? How does the Food and Drug Administration (FDA) approve medications for over-the-counter use?

What is the pathophysiology of a transient ischemic attack (TIA)? Who is at risk for a **TIA**?

What is the pathophysiology of **Wernicke-Korsakoff syndrome**? Who usually develops this syndrome? What is the treatment? What body system is affected?

Home Medications

☑ Self-Query: Possible Answers

Consult a drug text of choice to review the following:

Thiamine hydrochloride (B1) to decrease the possibility of Wernicke-Korsakoff syndrome.
Chlordiazepoxide hydrochloride (Librium) to decrease symptoms of withdrawal.
Lorazepam (Ativan) to decrease symptoms of withdrawal.
Oxazepam (Serax) to control agitation caused by alcohol withdrawal.

Body Systems

☑ Self-Query: Possible Answers

Neurological

Thiamine hydrochloride 100-mg tab daily
Chlordiazepoxide hydrochloride 25 mg 3 times a day orally
Lorazepam 1 mg orally, 1–2 every 2–4 hours as needed
Oxazepam 15 mg orally every 12 hours

Cardiovascular

Furosemide 40 mg every day orally
Potassium chloride 20 mEq every day orally
Nitro paste 1 inch every 6 hours topically
Thiamine hydrochloride 100-mg tab daily

Hematological

Thiamine hydrochloride 100-mg tab daily
Aspirin 325 mg orally daily
Cefpodoxime (Vantin) 200 mg twice a day orally

Pulmonary

Furosemide 40 mg every day orally
Potassium chloride 20 mEq every day orally
Nitro paste 1 inch every 6 hours topically

Gastrointestinal

Potassium chloride 20 mEq every day orally
Thiamine hydrochloride 100-mg tab daily
Aspirin 325 mg orally daily (are you aware of the affect it has in the stomach in regards to prostag-
    landins?)

Nutrition

Potassium chloride 20 mEq every day orally
Thiamine hydrochloride 100-mg tab daily

Genitourinary/renal

Potassium chloride 20 mEq every day orally
Furosemide 40 mg every day orally
Nitro paste 1 inch every 6 hours topically (think vasodilatation)

Aspirin 325 mg orally daily (think aspirin and renal impairment)
Cefpodoxime 200 mg twice a day orally

Musculoskeletal

Aspirin 325 mg orally daily (think aspirin and inflammation/antipyretic)

Endocrine

Although she has no medication specifically for this system, her other medications and substance abuse may affect her endocrine system.

Integumentary

Although there are no specific medications related to this system, be aware that any medication may affect it, particularly in a geriatric individual.

Immune

Although there are no specific medications related to this system, be aware that any medication may affect it, particularly in a geriatric individual.

Pain/comfort

Furosemide 40 mg every day orally (think edema discomfort)
Nitro paste 1 inch every 6 hours topically (think vasodilatation and chest pain)
Aspirin 325 mg orally daily (think aspirin and inflammation/antipyretic)

Physician Orders

0.9% NS at 125 mL/hr, given for hydration
Potassium chloride 40 mEq IV
Lab work reveals K+ 3.0
Flumazenil (Romazicon) 0.2 mg IV, given to reverse the possible overdose of benzodiazepines
Thiamine 100 mg IV, given for possible Wernicke-Korsakoff syndrome
Ciprofloxacin 400 mg IV every 12 hours
Review the foul odor from urine assessment

☑ Self-Query: Possible Answers

The patient had ingested an overdose of benzodiazepines with a large glass of wine. Because this was not known when she entered the emergency department, she was administered several interventions to reverse possible causes. If the physician suspected hypoglycemia, dextrose also would have been administered.

Case Study Inquiry

2

Vocabulary

❓ Self-Query

Before attempting to work the case study, define each of the vocabulary words. Although the words may have several subheadings, it will give you a place to begin your inquiry.

Angioedema
_____

Angiotensin-converting enzyme (ACE)
_____

Arteriovenous (AV) fistula
_____

Chronic obstructive pulmonary disease (COPD)
_____

Diabetic nephropathy
_____

End-stage renal failure (ESRF)
_____

Hemodialysis
_____

Hypertension
_____

Nephrosclerosis
_____

Phosphate binder
_____

Renin-angiotensin-aldosterone system (RAAS)
_____

Seizure
_____

Steal syndrome
_____

Type II diabetes
_____

You are completing a full assessment on a new patient admitted to your intensive care unit from the renal unit. He was transferred to the renal floor from the postanesthesia care unit (PACU) after surgery for a revision of a clotted AV fistula. He received hemodialysis 24 hours after surgery through a dual lumen hemodialysis graft, and within 5 minutes, he became unresponsive. Before you can finish a full assessment, he appears to have a seizure. Presently, all you know is the preceding information and that he is a 70-year-old black male. The patient's 35-year-old son is the only family member present. After interventions for the seizure activity, you continue the assessment and begin the medication reconciliation.

Recent History

The patient's history is given by the patient's 35-year-old son, who lives with him. The son verifies all the preceding information and states that the patient does not have a history of seizures. He also states that other than the worry about the need for the replacement of the AV fistula, there were no other concerns in the last week.

Home Medications

Albuterol (Proventil) 2.5 mg/3 mL (0.083% nebulizer solution) 2.5 mg every 4–6 hours

Amiodarone (Cordarone) tablet 200 mg twice daily with meals

Aspirin tablet 325 mg daily with breakfast

Bisoprolol (Zebeta) tablet 2.5 mg daily with breakfast

Budesonide (Pulmicort) 0.125 mg 2 times a day per nebulizer

Calcium carbonate (Os-Cal) 2 tabs every 12 hours

Digoxin (Lanoxin) tab 0.125 mg with breakfast

Epoetin SC injection 20,000 units Tuesday, Thursday, and Saturday

Esomeprazole (Nexium) capsule 40 mg daily

Ferrous sulfate 325 mg orally every 6 hours

Folic acid 1 mg orally daily

Gabapentin (Neurotin) capsule 300 mg twice daily

Insulin glargine (Lantus) 12 units SC injection at bedtime

Tramadol hydrochloride (Ultram) 100 mg extended release daily

? Self-Query

Using a drug book or pharmacology text that includes the mechanism of action, unlabeled uses, and pharmacokinetics for medications, answer the following questions. Make answers specific to this scenario.

What do I know about these medications? Do I know the recommended dose of, the recommended route for, and the best time of day to give these medications? Do I know what lab results I need regarding each medication? Do I know the approved use of each medication? Do I know the most common diseases treated by the listed medications? Are any off-label uses approved for each drug?

Albuterol

_____

_____

Amiodarone

_____

_____

Aspirin

_____

_____

Bisoprolol

_____

_____

Budesonide

_____

_____

Calcium carbonate

_____

_____

Digoxin

_____

_____

Epoetin

_____

_____

Esomeprazole

_____

_____

Ferrous sulfate

_____

_____

Folic acid

_____

_____

Gabapentin

_____

_____

Insulin glargine

_____

_____

Tramadol hydrochloride

_____

_____

Do I know the individual's past medical history by looking at the medication list?

_____

Allergies

ACE inhibitors

Self-Query

Do I know why ACE inhibitors are used?

_____

Do I know what the angiotensin-converting enzyme (ACE) does?

_____

Do I know the signs and symptoms of an adverse reaction to ACE?

_____

Do I know how this drug works?

_____

Body Systems

Self-Query

Be prepared to defend your answers.

Can I place each medication under the body system that it commonly affects?

Neurological

_____

Cardiovascular

_____

Hematological

_____

Pulmonary

_____

Gastrointestinal

_____

Nutrition

_____

Genitourinary/renal

_____

Musculoskeletal

_____

Endocrine

_____

Integumentary

_____

Immune

_____

Pain/comfort

_____

Mechanism of Action

Self-Query

Does the individual's medical history have an effect on the pharmacokinetics of each drug?

_____

_____

What contraindications do I need to address regarding the medications and this individual's health history?

_____

_____

Nursing Process

Self-Query

What nursing assessment will I do regarding each medication? What planning and implementation do I need to conduct for each medication? How do I evaluate each medication's effectiveness?

Albuterol

_____

Amiodarone

_____

Aspirin

_____

Bisoprolol

_____

Budesonide

_____

Calcium carbonate

_____

_____

Digoxin

_____

_____

Epoetin

_____

_____

Esomeprazole

_____

_____

Ferrous sulfate

_____

_____

Folic acid

_____

_____

Gabapentin

_____

_____

Insulin glargine

_____

_____

Tramadol hydrochloride

_____

_____

Do I need to be concerned with geriatric considerations for this individual?

_____

Physical Assessment Findings

Neurological Assessment

Opens eyes to verbal stimuli, follows verbal commands, minimal verbal response. Weak grips, plantar dorsiflexion and extension weak.

Cardiovascular and Hematological Assessment

Heart sounds S_1S_2 irregular; cardiac monitor reveals atrial fibrillation with frequent premature ventricular beats; distant heart sounds; radial pulses 1+ bilaterally; pedal pulses trace with noted trace edema to hands and feet. Blood pressure 102/50, skin warm and dry, capillary refill <3 seconds, new AV fistula to upper right arm, bruit and thrill present.

Pulmonary Assessment

Respiratory rate 16; decreased breath sounds throughout with expiratory wheezes and prolonged expiration; barrel chest noted; clubbing noted.

Gastrointestinal Assessment

Soft, nondistended abdomen; bowel sounds hypoactive in all quadrants.

Genitourinary Assessment

No urinary output.

Musculoskeletal Assessment

All extremities present with no deformities, bilaterally weak grips.

Endocrine Assessment

No exophthalmos, no slow-healing wounds, no goiter; noted history of diabetes.

Integumentary Assessment

Warm to touch; patches of dry skin; noted ecchymosis around site of previous AV fistula (left wrist); new AV fistula to upper right arm; thin, brittle nails.

Immune Assessment

No palpable lymph nodes.

Pain/Comfort Assessment

Son reports that client has pain in lower extremities and trouble buttoning shirts.

Physician Orders

Blood glucose monitoring before meals and at bedtime

Weigh every morning at 6:00

Lab: CBC/ FBS/Hgba1C

Blood pressure lying, sitting, and standing

Insulin regular (Novolin R insulin) for sliding scale

Dextrose 50% blood sugar < 40

Continue home medications

Nursing Process

Self-Query

What nursing assessment needs to be performed regarding each medication? What planning and implementation need to be conducted for each medication? How is each medication's effectiveness evaluated?

Insulin regular

_____

_____

_____

_____

Explain the physician's orders. Do any need clarification?

_____

_____

What possibly happened to the patient and why? Be specific.

_____

_____

_____

Synopsis

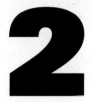

Because you can find answers to the self-queries in numerous texts, you will not find the answers to all of them here. However, you will find discussion of the individual case. The scenario relates to renal disease; therefore, purposefully look into the medication use and vocabulary as they relate to renal patients.

Vocabulary

When reviewing the vocabulary words, you might want to ask several questions: who, what, where, when, why, and how. This should give you a much broader understanding of each word.

Do yourself a favor and do not just give the shortest and simplest answer. The following questions are to be used as a guide. Instead of answering, "ACE inhibitors are a group of drugs that treat hypertension," ask:

Who is usually prescribed **angiotensin-converting enzyme (ACE)** inhibitors? Where is the ACE located? When are most prescribed? What medical diagnosis warrants an ACE inhibitor? How do they work?

☑ Self-Query: Possible Answers

When defining the remainder of the vocabulary words, ask the following questions:

Describe the pathophysiology behind **angioedema**. How are ACE inhibitors related to angioedema? What is the treatment for angioedema? What is the treatment for ACE-inhibitor-induced angioedema?

What is an **AV fistula**? Are there different types of fistulas? Where are they usually placed? Why are they used?

Describe the pathophysiology for **chronic obstructive pulmonary disease (COPD)**. Which diseases are included in COPD? Describe the differences between the underlying diseases in COPD. What is a primary risk factor for COPD?

What is the pathophysiology of **diabetic nephropathy**? If it is not treated, what can develop? What is the treatment? What body system(s) is affected?

What is the definition of **end-stage renal failure (ESRF)**? What is the pathophysiology behind ESRF? List three main causes of ESRF. Can the causes be prevented?

How does **hemodialysis** work? Who uses hemodialysis? How do we know that hemodialysis is working? Where can hemodialysis be administered? What is the pathophysiology behind seizures?

Does this man have essential (primary) and/or secondary **hypertension**? How did essential hypertension obtain its name? Which came first in this patient, the kidney disease or the hypertension? How will you explain your answer?

What is the pathophysiology of **nephrosclerosis**? What is the main cause of this disorder? Is there a treatment? What body system is affected?

What causes elevated phosphate levels? Who receives **phosphate binders**? What role does phosphorus play in the body? Why is phosphorus needed? What happens when there is too much phosphorus?

Describe the **renin-angiotensin-aldosterone system (RAAS)**. How do these systems regulate blood pressure and fluids in the body?

Can **seizures** be caused by altered calcium and phosphate levels? Does pH have a role in the seizure activity of a renal patient?

What is the definition of a **steal syndrome**? What is an example of a disease associated with steal syndrome? Are there different types of steal syndromes? If so, which type does this patient have?

What is the pathophysiology behind **type II diabetes**? How is it different from type I diabetes? Who is usually diagnosed with type II diabetes? Type I? Why is noninsulin-dependent diabetes mellitus (NIDDM) a misnomer for type II?

Body Systems

☑ Self-Query: Possible Answers

Neurological

> Gabapentin (Neurotin) capsule 300 mg 2 times a day
> Tramadol hydrochloride (Ultram) 100 mg extended release daily

Cardiovascular

> Amiodarone (Cordarone) tablet 200 mg twice daily with meals
> Aspirin tablet 325 mg daily with breakfast
> Bisoprolol (Zebeta) tablet 2.5 mg daily with breakfast
> Budesonide (Pulmicort) 0.125 mg 2 times a day per nebulizer (included here because of its effect on heart rate)
> Digoxin (Lanoxin) tab 0.125 mg with breakfast
> Epoetin SC injection 20,000 units, Tuesday, Thursday, and Saturday (included here because of the effect it has on blood pressure)

Hematological

> Aspirin tablet 325 mg daily with breakfast
> Calcium carbonate (Os-Cal) 2 tabs every 12 hours (used as a phosphate binder)
> Epoetin SC injection 20,000 units, Tuesday, Thursday, and Saturday
> Ferrous sulfate 325 mg orally every 6 hours
> Folic acid 1 mg orally daily

Pulmonary

> Albuterol (Proventil) 2.5 mg/3 mL (0.083% nebulizer solution) 2.5 mg every 4–6 hours
> Budesonide 0.125 mg 2 times a day per nebulizer
> Epoetin SC injection 20,000 units, Tuesday, Thursday, and Saturday (red blood cells [RBCs] and oxygenation)

Gastrointestinal

> Aspirin tablet 325 mg daily with breakfast (renal patients are prone to GI bleeds, and this also has an effect)
> Calcium carbonate 2 tabs every 12 hours (used here as a phosphate binder)
> Esomeprazole (Nexium) capsule 40 mg daily
> Ferrous sulfate 325 mg orally every 6 hours (may cause constipation)
> Tramadol hydrochloride 100 mg extended release daily (may cause constipation)

Nutrition

> Epoetin SC injection 20,000 units, Tuesday, Thursday, and Saturday
> Esomeprazole capsule 40 mg daily (may inhibit the uptake of folic acid and other nutrients depending on the time of dose)

Calcium carbonate 2 tabs every 12 hours
Ferrous sulfate 325 mg orally every 6 hours
Folic acid 1 mg orally daily
Insulin glargine (Lantus) 12 units SC injection at bedtime

Genitourinary/renal

Aspirin tablet 325 mg daily with breakfast (affects renal perfusion)
Calcium carbonate 2 tabs every 12 hours (used as a phosphate binder)
Epoetin SC injection 20,000 units, Tuesday, Thursday, and Saturday (promotes the production of
     RBC in the presence of renal failure)
Ferrous sulfate 325 mg orally every 6 hours
Folic acid 1 mg orally daily

Musculoskeletal

Calcium carbonate 2 tabs every 12 hours
Epoetin SC injection 20,000 units, Tuesday, Thursday, and Saturday
Ferrous sulfate 325 mg orally every 6 hours
Folic acid 1 mg orally daily
Tramadol hydrochloride 100 mg extended release daily

Endocrine

None

Integumentary

Calcium carbonate 2 tabs every 12 hours
Ferrous sulfate 325 mg orally every 6 hours
Folic acid 1 mg orally daily
Insulin glargine 12 units SC injection at bedtime
All are needed to assist in tissue repair and the prevention of skin breakdown.

Immune

Calcium carbonate 2 tabs every 12 hours
Epoetin SC injection 20,000 units, Tuesday, Thursday, and Saturday
Ferrous sulfate 325 mg orally every 6 hours
Folic acid 1 mg orally daily
Insulin glargine 12 units SC injection at bedtime
All are needed to assist in tissue repair and the prevention of skin breakdown.

Pain/comfort

Tramadol hydrochloride 100 mg extended release daily
Consider that the purpose of all the medications is to relieve symptoms that cause pain and
     discomfort.

Nursing Process

☑ Self Query: Possible Answers

The patient became hypovolemic during the hemodialysis, and his blood pressure dropped. He also
experienced disequilibrium syndrome.

Case Study Inquiry

3

Vocabulary

? Self-Query

Before attempting to work the case study, define each of the vocabulary words. Although the words may have several subheadings, it will give you a place to begin your inquiry.

Anemia

_____

Anticoagulation

_____

Atrial fibrillation

_____

Fatigue

_____

Garlic (allicin)

_____

Homocysteine

_____

International normalized ratio (INR)

_____

Off-label medication

_____

Platelet aggregation

_____

Prothrombin time (PT)

_____

Subdural hematoma

_____

Thrombus

_____

Triglycerides

_____

Vitamin K–dependent factors

_____

A 77-year-old female is brought to the emergency room after falling twice at her daughter's home. The first fall was in the bathtub, where she slipped while rising from the shower chair. She fell a second time when leaving her daughter's home to visit friends 2 hours later. Her daughter, who is present, states that her mother hit her head on the side of the house, and there is presently a large hematoma on the right side of her skull.

Recent History

The daughter states that her mother has been fatigued over the past 2 weeks and began taking an herbal remedy suggested by a friend. The daughter also states that her mother had complained about her arthritis "acting up." When the mother is further questioned, she states that she added garlic capsules to her daily medicines to help lower her cholesterol levels. The garlic is not on the list of home medications.

Home Medications

Aspirin 325 mg orally daily

Furosemide (Lasix) 40 mg orally daily

Metolazone (Zaroxolyn) 5 mg orally daily

Metoprolol succinate (Toprol-XL) 50 mg orally daily

Potassium (K-DUR) orally 20 mEq daily

Rosuvastatin calcium (Crestor) 10 mg orally daily

Warfarin (Coumadin) 5 mg orally daily

Now add:

Garlic 2 capsules every morning

♀ Self-Query

Using a drug book or pharmacology text that contains the mechanism of action, unlabeled uses, and pharmacokinetics for medications, answer the following questions. Make answers specific to this scenario.

What do I know about these medications? Do I know the recommended dose of, the recommended route for, and the best time of day to give these medications? Do I know what lab results I need regarding each medication? Do I know the approved use of each medication? Do I know the most common diseases treated by the listed medications? Are any off-label uses approved for each drug?

Aspirin

_____

_____

Furosemide

_____

_____

Metolazone

_____

_____

Metoprolol succinate

_____

_____

Potassium

_____

_____

Rosuvastatin calcium

_____

_____

Warfarin

_____

_____

Garlic capsule

_____

_____

Do I know the individual's past medical history by looking at the medication list?

_____

_____

Allergies

Codeine

Morphine

Self-Query

Do I know why codeine and morphine are used?

_____

Do I know the signs and symptoms of an adverse reaction to codeine and morphine?

_____

How are these medications similar and how are they different?

_____

Body Systems

Self-Query

Be prepared to defend your answers.

Can I place each medication under the body system that it commonly affects?

Neurological

_____

Cardiovascular

_____

Hematological

_____

Pulmonary

_____

Gastrointestinal

_____

Nutrition

_____

Genitourinary/renal

_____

Musculoskeletal

_____

Endocrine

_____

Integumentary

_____

Immune

_____

Pain/comfort

_____

Mechanism of Action

☝ Self-Query

Does the individual's medical history have an effect on the pharmacokinetics of each drug?

_____

_____

What contraindications do I need to address regarding the medications and medical history?

_____

_____

Nursing Process

☝ Self-Query

What nursing assessment will I perform regarding each medication? What is a priority nursing diagnosis regarding each medication? What planning and implementation do I need to do for each medication? How do I evaluate each medication's effectiveness?

Aspirin

_____

_____

Furosemide

_____

_____

Metolazone

_____

_____

Metoprolol succinate

_____

_____

Potassium

_____

_____

Rosuvastatin calcium

_____

_____

Warfarin

_____

_____

Garlic capsule

_____

_____

Do I need to be concerned about geriatric considerations with this individual?

_____

Physical Assessment Findings
Neurological Assessment

Alert and oriented; no acute distress; reports headache; pupils equal, bilateral cataract removal noted; presently a large hematoma on the right forehead with bruising on the right side of the face; cranial nerves II–XII intact. No focal defects.

Cardiovascular and Hematological Assessment

Atrial fibrillation 88 beats per monitor, no carotid bruits, no JVD, S_1S_2 upon auscultation, mild edema to ankles, pulses intact to lower extremities, blood pressure 90/60, capillary refill at 3 seconds. T. 99.6°F, PT 80, INR 5, K+ 3.0. Na+ 128.

Pulmonary Assessment

Breath sounds clear; respirations even, unlabored.

Gastrointestinal and Nutrition Assessment

Dentures; eats without problems; small-framed black woman; weight 110 pounds; colonoscopy last week, no problems.

Genitourinary/Renal Assessment

Slightly incontinent; wears briefs; no noted trace hematuria in urinalysis.

Musculoskeletal Assessment

Mild osteoarthritis; reports being stiff but continues to work in her garden; slight limited range of motion.

Endocrine Assessment

No exophthalmos; no slow-healing wounds; no goiter; skin warm and dry.

Integumentary Assessment

Several areas of bruising appearing after admission to emergency room (facial, hip, and right shoulder).

Immune Assessment

No palpable lymph nodes.

Pain/Comfort Assessment

Noted headache and tenderness to right hip, right thigh.

Physician Orders

Stop garlic
Stop warfarin
0.9% NS at 100mL/hr
Potassium chloride 40 mEq IV
Phytonadione (Aquamephyton) 5 mg IM now
CT scan
Consult to neurological intensive care

Self-Query

Why is garlic stopped?

_____

_____

Why is warfarin stopped?

_____

_____

What is the classification of each medication? How is each medication usually given? Why did the physician order each medication for this individual?

Potassium chloride

_____

_____

Phytonadione

_____

_____

Nursing Process

? Self-Query

What do I think happened to this individual and why? (Be specific.)

_____

_____

_____

Synopsis

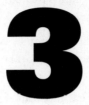

3

Because you can find answers to the self-queries in numerous texts, you will not find the answers to all of them here. However, you will find discussion of the individual case. The scenario relates to geriatrics and anticoagulants; therefore, purposefully look into the medication use and vocabulary as they relate to these patients and this issue.

Vocabulary

When reviewing the vocabulary words, you might want to ask several questions: who, what, where, when, why, and how. This should give you a much broader understanding of each word.

Do yourself a favor and do not just give the shortest and simplest answer. Use the following example for garlic: Instead of answering, "Garlic belongs in the onion family," ask:

Who benefits from ingesting **garlic**? What is the compound in garlic that is thought to be beneficial? Where can garlic be obtained? When is it not a good idea to use garlic? Why do some patients benefit, or think they benefit, from garlic?

☑ Self-Query: Possible Answers

When defining the remainder of the vocabulary words, ask the following questions:

What is the definition of **anemia**? Is anemia a disease or a symptom? What type of anemia does the patient in the case study possibly suffer from? Is there a connection between some of this individual's medications and the anemia? Explain.

What is the pathophysiology of **anticoagulation**? What medication(s) is being taken by the patient that alters anticoagulation? How is anticoagulation measured? What does it reveal? Does it need to be high or low?

What is the pathophysiology behind **atrial fibrillation**? How is it different from a sinus rhythm? Who is at risk for A-fib? What medications are related to the control of the rhythm?

What causes **fatigue**? Who experiences fatigue? How is fatigue different from being tired? How is fatigue treated?

How does **homocysteine** affect the vascular system? Where is it found in our diets? Do we need a high level or a low level? What vitamins are needed to lower the homocysteine levels?

What is an **international normalized ratio (INR)**? Why is it measured? What medication(s) is being taken by the patient that alters the INR? How is it measured? What does it reveal? Are the values different for different diagnoses?

What does **"off label"** mean in regard to medications?

Give an example of a **platelet aggregation**. Why is it needed? What causes platelets to aggregate? What medication(s) is the patient taking that will affect her platelets? How long does a platelet live?

What is a **prothrombin time (PT)**? Why is it measured? What medication(s) is being taken by the individual that alters the PT? How is it measured? What does it reveal? Does it need to be high or low?

What is the pathophysiology of a **thrombus**? Is there a difference between arterial and venous clots? Who is at risk for a thrombus? How is a thrombus treated?

What role do **triglycerides** play in the body? How is an excess of triglycerides harmful?

What is the pathophysiology for a **subdural hematoma**? After reading the scenario, did this patient have a subdural hematoma? Do you have enough information to decide? Did the medications play a part in this woman's hematoma? Which medications contributed to the INR of 5?

What is **vitamin K**? Why is it needed? What medication(s) being taken by this individual can be altered by vitamin K?

Body Systems

☑ Self-Query: Possible Answers

Neurological

Any of these medications can be detrimental neurologically in the geriatric individual.

Cardiovascular

Aspirin 325 mg orally daily
Furosemide (Lasix) 40 mg orally daily
Garlic 2 capsules every morning
Rosuvastatin calcium (Crestor) 10 mg orally daily
Metolazone (Zaroxolyn) 5 mg orally daily
Metoprolol succinate (Toprol-XL) 50 mg orally daily
Potassium (K-DUR) orally 20 mEq daily
Warfarin (Coumadin) 5 mg orally daily

Hematological

Aspirin 325 mg orally daily
Furosemide 40 mg orally daily
Garlic 2 capsules every morning
Metolazone 5 mg orally daily
Metoprolol succinate 50 mg orally daily
Phytonadione (Aquamephyton) 5 mg IM now
Potassium orally 20 mEq daily
Rosuvastatin calcium 10 mg orally daily
Warfarin 5 mg orally daily

Pulmonary

None

Gastrointestinal

Any of the following medications can detrimentally alter the gastrointestinal tract in the geriatric individual:
Aspirin 325 mg orally daily
Garlic 2 capsules every morning
Rosuvastatin calcium 10 mg orally daily
Warfarin 5 mg orally daily

Nutrition

Be aware that this geriatric individual will most likely have nutritional deficits. This will alter protein binding and the levels of the medications available in the patient's system.

Garlic 2 capsules every morning
Potassium orally 20 mEq daily
Rosuvastatin calcium 10 mg orally daily

Genitourinary/renal

Be aware that this geriatric individual will most likely have some age-related decreased renal function. This will alter excretion and the levels of the medications remaining in the system.

Aspirin 325 mg orally daily—will alter prostaglandins in the kidneys needed to assist in profusion
Furosemide 40 mg orally daily
Metolazone 5 mg orally daily

Musculoskeletal

Any of these medications can alter this system in the geriatric individual.

Integumentary

Any of these medications can alter this system in the geriatric individual.

Immune

Any of these medications can alter this system in the geriatric individual.

Pain/comfort

Any of these medications can be detrimental in the geriatric individual. Consider that all the medications are to relieve symptoms that cause pain and discomfort. No analgesics were prescribed, however, and many patients will not list OTC medications.

Nursing Process

☑ Self-Query: Possible Answers

The patient stated in the scenario that her arthritis was "acting up," but she did not reveal what she took. More than likely, she took Tylenol ES or another form of aspirin. The garlic she took to help lower her cholesterol has been shown to interact with the other anticoagulants and elevate the clotting factors. She should not have started the garlic without consulting her healthcare provider. This emphasizes that we in the healthcare profession should spend more time educating the public on the use of herbs and over-the-counter medications in combination with prescription medications.

Crestor is also known to elevate the PT/INR.

Case Study Inquiry

4

Vocabulary

? Self-Query

Before attempting to work the case study, define each of the vocabulary words. Although the words may have several subheadings, it will give you a place to begin your inquiry.

Autoimmune diseases
_____

Culture and sensitivity (C&S)
_____

Immunocompromised
_____

Methicillin-resistant *Staphylococcus aureus* **(MRSA)**
_____

Podiatrist
_____

Pseudomonas
_____

Rheumatoid arthritis
_____

Rheumatologist
_____

Serous drainage
_____

Sleep apnea
_____

Thrombocytopenia
_____

Wound stages
_____

You are assessing a client visiting the clinic today. She is 56 years old but appears much older. She is frail and looks to be about 5'7" and 110 pounds. She had a culture and sensitivity (C&S) collected on a wound on her lower left leg 3 days ago. The healthcare provider prescribed vancomycin, but after the first dose, the client became red and flushed and was switched to a different antibiotic. She returns today to receive the results of methicillin-resistant *staphylococcus aureus* (MRSA).

Recent History

The client recently scraped her leg on a bike pedal while riding in her neighborhood. She noticed what appeared to be a small pimple 2 days later on the spot where she scraped her leg. She placed a dressing over the area. She removed the dressing 2 days later hoping that the spot had healed, but it had increased in size and was draining. She called the clinic.

Home Medications

Celecoxib (Celebrex) 200-mg capsule orally daily

Fentanyl 75-mcg patch, change every 3 days

Hydroxychloroquin (Plaquenil) 200-mg tab orally daily

Meropenem (Merrem) 2 g IV every 8 hours (delivered per home health and an infusion company)

Omeprazole (Prilosec) 20 mg delayed release orally daily

Oxycodone (OxyIR) 5-mg tab as needed for breakthrough pain

Oxycodone hydrochloride 10-mg tab orally every 12 hours

Prednisone 2-mg tab orally daily

Self-Query

Using a drug book or pharmacology text that contains the mechanism of action, unlabeled uses, and pharmacokinetics for medications, answer the following questions. Make answers specific to this scenario.

What do I know about these medications? Do I know the recommended dose of, the recommended route for, and the best time of day to give these medications? Do I know what lab results I need regarding each medication? Do I know the approved use of each medication? Do I know the most common diseases treated by the listed medications? Are any off-label uses approved for each drug?

Celecoxib

_____

_____

Fentanyl

_____

_____

Hydroxychloroquin

_____

_____

Meropenem

_____

_____

Omeprazole

_____

_____

Oxycodone

_____

_____

Oxycodone hydrochloride

_____

_____

Prednisone

_____

_____

Do I know the individual's past medical history by looking at the medication list?

_____

_____

Do I know the serious toxicity of taking hydroxychloroquin?

_____

Allergies

The patient states that she had "flushing of skin" when given vancomycin before the culture was obtained.

Self-Query

Do I know why vancomycin is used?

_____

Do I know the signs and symptoms of an adverse reaction to vancomycin?

_____

Do I know what red man syndrome looks like?

_____

Body Systems

Self-Query

Be prepared to defend your answers.

Can I place each medication under the body system that it commonly affects?

Neurological

_____

Cardiovascular

_____

Hematological

_____

Pulmonary

_____

Gastrointestinal

_____

Nutrition

_____

Genitourinary/renal

_____

Musculoskeletal

_____

Endocrine

_____

Integumentary

_____

Immune

_____

Pain/comfort

_____

Mechanism of Action

? Self-Query

Does the individual's medical history have an effect on the pharmacokinetics of each drug?

_____

_____

What contraindications do I need to address regarding the medications and medical history?

_____

_____

Nursing Process

? Self-Query

What nursing assessment will I perform regarding each medication? What planning and implementation do I need to conduct for each medication? How do I evaluate each medication's effectiveness?

Celecoxib

_____

Fentanyl

_____

Hydroxychloroquin

_____

Meropenem

_____

Omeprazole

_____

Oxycodone

_____

Oxycodone hydrochloride

_____

Prednisone

Do I need to be concerned with geriatric considerations with this individual?

Physical Assessment Findings

Neurological Assessment

Pupils equal, round, and reactive to light. Speech clear, appropriate.

Cardiovascular and Hematological Assessment

BNP negative, K+ 3.0, S_1S_2 monitor reveals sinus of 50.
Blood pressure 90/50, no edema, extremities pale, capillary refill at 3 seconds.
Bruising to upper extremities and bruising noted on shins bilaterally.

Pulmonary Assessment

Lungs clear throughout with respiratory rate 12 per minute.

Gastrointestinal Assessment

Positive bowel sounds, poor dentations, diarrhea last 24 hours.

Genitourinary Assessment

Denies problems.

Musculoskeletal Assessment

Noted stiffness in movements; elevated C-reactive protein (CRP); erythrocyte sedimentation rate (ESR) elevated; noted round, movable, and nontender subcutaneous nodules on fingers and elbows.

Endocrine Assessment

No exophthalmia, no hirsutism, no goiter.

Integumentary Assessment

Bruising to upper extremities and bruising noted to left lower extremity. Open wound to left lower extremity. Noted open subcutaneous nodule below open wound, red and draining at present. IV site to right antecubital 0.9% NS.

Immune Assessment

No palpable lymph nodes.

Pain/Comfort Assessment

Pain with movement, tenderness to joints and wound area.

Physician Orders

Stop meropenem

Restart vancomycin 1 g every 12 hours, infuse over one and a half hours and no quicker administer diphenhydramine 30 minutes before infusion

Consult infectious disease

Consult wound care nurse

Admit and continue home meds

Self-Query

Why stop meropenem? What classification is meropenem?

_____

_____

Why restart the vancomycin? What classification is vancomycin? How is it given?

_____

_____

Nursing Process

Self-Query

What nursing interventions are used?

_____

_____

What labs are drawn?

_____

_____

What happened to the patient and why? Be specific.

_____

_____

_____

Synopsis

4

Because you can find answers to the self-queries in numerous texts, you will not find the answers to all of them here. However, you will find discussion of the individual case. The scenario relates to autoimmune consequences; therefore, purposefully look into the medication use and vocabulary as they relate to autoimmune patients.

Vocabulary

When reviewing the vocabulary words, you might want to ask several questions: who, what, where, when, why, and how. This should give you a much broader understanding of each word.

Do yourself a favor and do not just give the shortest and simplest answer. Use the example of immuncompromised as a guide. Instead of answering, "Immunocompromised refers to a person's immune system being compromised" (which, by the way, is not the proper way to define a word; never use the word being defined in its own definition), ask:

Who is at risk for being **immunocompromised**? What is the pathophysiology behind being immuno-compromised? When is being immunocompromised most dangerous? Why do certain medications place a person at risk for being immunocompromised?

☑ Self-Query: Possible Answers

When defining the remainder of the vocabulary words, ask the following questions:

What is the definition of an **autoimmune disease**? Who is at risk for these types of diseases?

What are the benefits of performing a **culture and sensitivity (C&S)** on a specimen? What is the time frame for a C&S? What does a colony count in the C&S reveal? Why is the bacteria type important? Why is susceptibility testing important in the choice of the medication?

What caused the development of **methicillin-resistant *Staphylococcus aureus* (MRSA)** in our society? Who is at greatest risk for MRSA? In the scenario, the patient was prescribed vancomycin. Was this appropriate?

What does a **podiatrist** do? What disorders will this specialist see? Why would the person in this scenario be seeing this specialist? Which medications might this specialist have prescribed?

What type of organism is **pseudomonas**? Where is a person most likely to acquire pseudomonas? When is a person most at risk for acquiring pseudomonas? How does it affect the immunocompro-mised person?

What is the pathophysiology behind **rheumatoid arthritis (RA)**? Who is at risk for RA? How is the pathophysiology different for osteoarthritis? How are the treatments different? How are the symptoms different?

What does a **rheumatologist** do? What disorders will this specialist see? Why would the person in this scenario be seeing this specialist? Which medications might this specialist have prescribed?

What role does **serous drainage** play in healing? What products are located in serous fluid?

What is the pathophysiology behind **sleep apnea**? How does it alter immunity? How is it treated?

What is the pathophysiology behind **thrombocytopenia**? Who is at risk for thrombocytopenia? In this scenario, are there any medications that can induce thrombocytopenia? How is it detected? What are the treatments? Which body systems are altered in thrombocytopenia?

What **stage wound** does the patient in this scenario have? How are wounds staged? How has the immunocompromised state of this individual altered the healing process? What does a wound require to heal?

Body Systems

☑ Self-Query: Possible Answers

Neurological

> Oxycodone hydrochloride 10-mg tab orally every 12 hours
> Fentanyl 75-mcg patch, change every 3 days
> Oxycodone (OxyIR) 5-mg tab PRN for breakthrough pain
> Hydroxychloroquin (Plaquenil) 200-mg tab orally daily (can alter sensory perception in some cases)

Cardiovascular

> None

Hematological

> (Placed here to stress the effect these medications have on this system.)
> Hydroxychloroquin 200-mg tab orally daily
> Prednisone 2-mg tab orally daily
> Meropenem (Merrem) 2 g IV every 8 hours
> Vancomycin discontinued

Pulmonary

> (Placed here to stress the effect that these medications have on this system; at first may cause decreased respiratory effort.)
> Oxycodone hydrochloride 10-mg tab orally every 12 hours
> Fentanyl 75-mcg patch, change every 3 days
> Oxycodone 5-mg tab as needed for breakthrough pain

Gastrointestinal

> (Several medications placed here to stress the effect that these medications have on this system.)
> Celecoxib (Celebrex) 200-mg capsule orally daily
> Hydroxychloroquin 200-mg tab orally daily
> Omeprazole (Prilosec) 20 mg delayed release orally daily
> Prednisone 2-mg tab orally daily
> Oxycodone hydrochloride 10-mg tab orally every 12 hours
> Fentanyl 75-mcg patch, change every 3 days
> Oxycodone 5-mg tab as needed for breakthrough pain

Nutrition

> Omeprazole 20 mg delayed release orally daily
> Prednisone 2-mg tab orally daily

Genitourinary/renal

(Several medications placed here to stress the effect that these medications have on this system.)
Celecoxib 200-mg capsule orally daily
Fentanyl 75-mcg patch, change every 3 days
Hydroxychloroquin 200-mg tab orally daily
Meropenem 2 g IV every 8 hours
Omeprazole 20 mg delayed release orally daily
Oxycodone 5-mg tab as needed for breakthrough pain
Oxycodone hydrochloride 10-mg tab orally every 12 hours
Prednisone 2-mg tab orally daily
Vancomycin discontinued

Musculoskeletal

Celecoxib 200-mg capsule orally daily
Hydroxychloroquin 200-mg tab orally daily
Prednisone 2-mg tab orally daily

Integumentary

Hydroxychloroquin 200-mg tab orally daily
Prednisone 2-mg tab orally daily

Immune

(Several medications placed here to stress the effect these medications have on this system.)
Hydroxychloroquin 200-mg tab orally daily
Prednisone 2-mg tab orally daily
Meropenem 2 g IV every 8 hours
Vancomycin discontinued

Pain/comfort

Celecoxib 200-mg capsule orally daily
Fentanyl 75-mcg patch, change every 3 days
Hydroxychloroquin 200-mg tab orally daily
Meropenem 2 g IV every 8 hours
Omeprazole 20 mg delayed release orally daily
Oxycodone 5-mg tab as needed for breakthrough pain
Oxycodone hydrochloride 10-mg tab orally every 12 hours
Prednisone 2-mg tab orally daily
Vancomycin discontinued
Consider that all the medications are to relieve symptoms that cause pain and discomfort.

Nursing Process

☑ Self-Query: Possible Answers

The patient experienced red man syndrome, which is common with rapid infusions of vancomycin. The vancomycin infusion can be restarted. Most patients may receive antihistamine medications before the drug is restarted, as was the case with this patient. The patient was pretreated with acetaminophen and diphenhydramine and then was infused at a much slower rate. Several medications given for the RA decreased her ability to heal and, in fact, caused her to be immunocompromised.

The following medications are used as an anti-inflammatory and may decrease the individual's ability to fight infection:

Hydroxychloroquin 200-mg tab orally daily
Prednisone 2-mg tab orally daily

The patient was placed back on vancomycin because she was to receive IV therapy at home. The pharmacist considered the stability and ease of infusion for both medications. Vancomycin was recommended as a cheaper and effective alternative to meropenem.

Case Study Inquiry

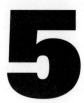

Vocabulary

Self-Query

Before attempting to work the case study, define the vocabulary words. Although the words may have several subheadings, it will give you a place to begin your inquiry.

Autoimmune diseases
_____

Bowel incontinence
_____

Dysphasia
_____

Hepatic encephalopathy
_____

Hyperglycemia
_____

Hyperlipidemia
_____

Inflammation (include stages and major blood components)
_____

Inflammatory cardiomyopathy
_____

Kyphosis
_____

Multiple sclerosis
_____

Myasthenia gravis
_____

Myopathy: polymyositis (PM)
_____

Occupational therapy
_____

Osteoporosis
_____

Panniculitis

You are interviewing a 62-year-old female. She is 5′4″. Over a period of 2–3 weeks, she noticed that she would have difficulty lifting her granddaughter into the air to play. She thought that maybe the child was just growing bigger. Today, she noticed that she could not place dishes on the top shelf in her kitchen; she stated that her arms "would not move." She noticed that when she walked up a flight of stairs yesterday for exercise, her hips and thighs did not seem to want to work very well either. Her son has brought her to the clinic.

Recent History

The patient states that she has always been mostly healthy. She has a new grandchild and has had no recent cold or virus that she can remember. The only new medication that she remembers is Tagamet (cimetidine). She is worried that she may have multiple sclerosis. Her son had placed all her present medications in a bag, which she brought with her.

Home Medications

Aspirin (Ecotrin) 325 mg orally daily

Cimetidine (Tagamet) 300 mg 4 times a day orally

Diltiazem hydrochloride (Cardizem) 120 mg daily orally

Ferrous sulfate 1 tab daily orally

Levothyroxine sodium (Synthroid) 112 mcg daily orally

Sulfamethoxazole and trimethoprim (abbreviated TMP-SMZ; trade name: Bactrim) 1 tab every 12 hours for 7 days (2 tabs remaining)

Tolterodine tartrate (Detrol) 2 mg twice a day orally

☞ Self-Query

Using a drug book or pharmacology text that contains the mechanism of action, unlabeled uses, and pharmacokinetics for medications, answer the following questions. Make answers specific to this scenario.

What do I know about these medications? Do I know the recommended dose of, the recommended route for, and the best time of day to give these medications? Do I know what lab results I need regarding each medication? Do I know the approved use of each medication? Do I know the most common diseases treated by the listed medications? Are any off-label uses approved for each drug?

Aspirin

_____

_____

Cimetidine

_____

_____

Diltiazem hydrochloride

_____

_____

Ferrous sulfate

_____

_____

Levothyroxine sodium

_____

_____

TMP-SMZ

_____

_____

Tolterodine tartrate

_____

_____

Do I know the individual's past medical history by looking at the medication list?

_____

_____

Why should you query her on the Bactrim, and would you consider it a routine home medication? Explain your answer.

_____

_____

Allergies

The patient states that she is allergic to sulfa.

Self-Query

Why should this allergy be further investigated?

_____

Do I know the signs and symptoms of an adverse reaction to sulfa?

_____

Body Systems

Self-Query

Be prepared to defend your answers .

Can I place each medication under the body system that it commonly affects?

Neurological

_____

Cardiovascular

_____

Hematological

_____

Pulmonary

_____

Gastrointestinal

_____

Nutrition

_____

Genitourinary/renal

_____

Musculoskeletal

_____

Endocrine

_____

Integumentary

_____

Immune

_____

Pain/comfort

_____

Nursing Process

Self-Query

What nursing assessment will I perform regarding each medication? What planning and implementation do I need for each medication? How do I evaluate each medication's effectiveness?

Aspirin

_____

_____

Cimetidine

_____

_____

Diltiazem hydrochloride

_____

_____

Ferrous sulfate

_____

_____

Levothyroxine sodium

_____

_____

TMP-SMZ

_____

_____

Tolterodine tartrate

_____

_____

Do I need to be concerned with geriatric considerations with this individual?

_____

Physical Assessment Findings

Neurological Assessment

Alert, oriented, speech clear, grips weak bilaterally, gait uneven.

Cardiovascular and Hematological Assessment

BNP negative, K+ 3.9, S_1S_2 monitor reveals sinus of 90.

Blood pressure 146/80, no edema, capillary refill at 3 seconds.

Bruising to upper extremities. Patient stated that her stools were dark.

No pericardial rub noted, no chest pain.

Pulmonary Assessment

Clear to auscultation.

Gastrointestinal Assessment

Hyperactive bowel sounds; no dentures, has own teeth.

Genitourinary Assessment

Voided for urine specimen/strong odor.

Musculoskeletal Assessment

Weakness to muscles of the hips and thighs, upper arms. Weakness in shrugging shoulder. Gait uneven. No difficulty swallowing. No recent weight loss. Noted tenderness to hands and hip and thigh areas. Unable to raise from lying position without assistance.

Endocrine Assessment

No exophthalmia, no hirsutism, no slow-healing wounds, no goiter.

Integumentary Assessment

Bruising to upper extremities. IV site to right antecubital 0.9% NS. Purplish rash on face and neck.

Immune Assessment

No palpable lymph nodes.

Pain/Comfort Assessment

Muscle tenderness and joint pain.

Physician Orders

Lab: ANA, ESR; MRI, EMG; T_3 and T_4.

Stop TMP-SMZ.

Urine culture and sensitivity (C&S).

Calcium citrate (Citracal) 2 tabs daily with breakfast.

Prednisone 2 mg every 6 hours will be given depending on results of the tests.

Self-Query

What does the physician suspect?

_____

_____

What is the classification of each medication? Why is it usually prescribed? Why was it prescribed for this patient? How is each medication administered?

Calcium citrate

_____

_____

Prednisone

_____

_____

Why would the physician stop the TMP-SMZ and order a C&S of the urine?

_____

_____

What do you think was the final diagnosis?

_____

_____

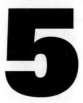

Because you can find answers to the self-queries in numerous texts, you will not find the answers to all of them here. However, you will find discussion of the individual case. The scenario relates to autoimmune disorders; therefore, purposefully look into the medication use and vocabulary as they relate to autoimmune patients.

Vocabulary

When reviewing the vocabulary words, you might want to ask several questions: who, what, where, when, why, and how. This should give you a much broader understanding of each word.

Do yourself a favor and do not just give the shortest and simplest answer. Use the following example for palliative care: Instead of answering, "Palliative care is special care focused on the pain experienced during a chronic or terminal illness," ask:

Why would a person with an autoimmune disorder need this type of **palliative care**? Where is this type of care most likely to be given? When is this type of care needed? Who is eligible for this type of care? How is this different from hospice care? How is it similar to hospice care? What types of medications are used in palliative care?

☑ Self-Query: Possible Answers

When defining the remainder of the vocabulary words, ask the following questions:

What are the causes of **bowel incontinence**? What are the medications used to treat bowel incontinence? Who is at risk for bowel incontinence? Is it considered a symptom of a disease or medication induced? Which autoimmune diseases cause bowel incontinence?

What is **dysphasia**? What commonly causes dysphasia? Is it medication/disease induced? Who is at risk for dysphasia? What are the medication treatments for dysphasia? Is this something that a person with certain types of autoimmune disorders might develop?

What is the pathophysiology of **hepatic encephalopathy**? Who develops hepatic encephalopathy? What is the medication treatment? What body system is affected? Is it an autoimmune disorder?

What is the pathophysiology of **hyperglycemia**? What commonly causes hyperglycemia? Why might certain medications induce hyperglycemia? How are people with autoimmune diseases affected?

What is the pathophysiology of **hyperlipidemia**? Who is at risk for hyperlipidemia? What commonly causes hyperlipidemia? Is it medication/disease induced? Is there a medication treatment for this?

What is the pathophysiology for **inflammation**? What commonly causes inflammation? What lab test is ordered to assess for inflammation? Is it medication/disease induced? Who is at risk for inflammation? What are the medication treatments for inflammation?

What is the pathophysiology of **inflammatory cardiomyopathy**? Who develops this disorder? What is the medication treatment? What body system is affected? How would this be classified as an autoimmune disorder?

What is the pathophysiology of **kyphosis**? Who is at risk for kyphosis? Where is kyphosis seen? Is there a medication treatment for kyphosis?

What is the pathophysiology of **multiple sclerosis (MS)**? Who develops MS? What is the medication treatment? What body system is affected? Is it an autoimmune disorder?

What is the pathophysiology of **myasthenia gravis**? Who develops myasthenia gravis? What is the medication treatment? What body system is affected? Is it an autoimmune disorder?

What commonly causes **myopathy**? Is it medication/disease induced? Who is at risk for myopathy? What are the medication treatments for myopathy?

What is **occupational therapy (OT)**? Who benefits from OT? How would OT benefit someone with an autoimmune disease? How is it different from physical therapy?

What is the pathophysiology of **osteoporosis**? Who is at risk for osteoporosis? When is osteoporosis most commonly seen? Is it medication/disease induced? What are the medication treatments for osteoporosis? What is the difference between osteoporosis and osteoarthritis? What are the medications used for osteoporosis?

What is the pathophysiology of **panniculitis**? Who usually develops panniculitis? What is the treatment? What body system is affected? Why might a person with an autoimmune disorder develop panniculitis?

Body Systems

☑ Self-Query: Possible Answers

Neurological

> Aspirin (Ecotrin) 325 mg orally daily
> Tolterodine tartrate (Detrol) 2 mg twice a day orally
> The drug works by blocking the nerve impulses that prompt the bladder to contract.

Cardiovascular

> Diltiazem hydrochloride (Cardizem) 120 mg daily orally
> Levothyroxine sodium (Synthroid) 112 mcg daily orally (Levothyroxine sodium is not a cardiac drug, but it is placed here to remind you that problems with the thyroid have an effect on the cardiac system.)
> Aspirin 325 mg orally daily (placed here because of the antiplatelet effects of the medications)

Hematological

> Aspirin 325 mg orally daily
> Ferrous sulfate 1 tab daily orally
> Sulfamethoxazole and trimethoprim (abbreviated TMP-SMZ; trade name: Bactrim) 1 tab every 12 hours for 7 days (2 tabs remaining)

Pulmonary

> None

Gastrointestinal

> Aspirin 325 mg orally daily (This medication is enteric coated and should cause no harm to the GI system because it is altered in the small intestine.)
> Cimetidine (Tagamet) 300 mg 4 times a day orally
> Ferrous sulfate 1 tab daily orally (major effect is constipation)
> Levothyroxine sodium 112 mcg daily orally (Although the medication targets the thyroid, the GI system is altered when the thyroid is not functioning.)

Genitourinary/renal

Aspirin 325 mg orally daily (alters the prostaglandins in the kidneys)

Ferrous sulfate 1 tab daily orally

Tolterodine tartrate 2 mg twice a day orally

TMP-SMZ 1 tab every 12 hours for 7 days, 2 tabs remaining. (This medication is commonly used for UTIs.)

Musculoskeletal

Aspirin 325 mg orally daily

Levothyroxine sodium 112 mcg daily orally

Calcium citrate (Citracal) 2 tabs daily

Tolterodine tartrate 2 mg twice a day orally

Endocrine

Levothyroxine sodium 112 mcg daily orally (focuses on the thyroid gland)

Prednisone 2 mg (raises glucose levels)

Integumentary

Prednisone 2 mg

Immune

TMP-SMZ 1 tab every 12 hours for 7 days, 2 tabs remaining

Prednisone 2 mg (alters the body's ability to fight infection)

Pain/comfort

These medications are not classified as pain medications; however, they are given to decrease the pain and discomfort of certain disease processes.

Aspirin 325 mg orally daily—can be used for pain but is taken daily as an antiplatelet medication

Cimetidine 300 mg 4 times a day orally—taken for GI distress (possible esophagitis)

Diltiazem hydrochloride 120 mg daily orally—taken to decrease the distress caused by hypertension, angina, and certain heart rhythm disorders

Ferrous sulfate 1 tab daily orally—taken to decrease the distress caused by iron-deficiency anemia

Levothyroxine sodium 112 mcg daily orally—taken to decrease the distress caused by thyroid disorders

TMP-SMZ 1 tab every 12 hours for 7 days, 2 tabs remaining—taken to decrease the distress caused by bladder infection (The history of bladder incontinence may be a risk factor for UTI.)

Tolterodine tartrate 2 mg twice a day orally—taken to decrease the distress caused by bladder disorders such as frequent urination, urgency, and urge incontinence

Nursing Process

☑ Self-Query: Possible Answers

The sulfa allergy should be further investigated because TMP-SMZ is a combination of sulfamethoxazole (sulfa) and trimethoprim. The bruising was also an indication that the patient had balance problems. She was diagnosed with multiple sclerosis and placed on prednisone. The prednisone was prescribed to help reduce the inflammation in the brain and spinal cord. It is used to accelerate recovery between episodes and, it is hoped, to lessen the symptoms experienced in MS. The patient was referred to a neurologist and placed in a clinical trial for MS.

Case Study Inquiry

6

Vocabulary

Self-Query

Before attempting to work the case study, define each of the vocabulary words. Although the words may have several subheadings, it will give you a place to begin your inquiry.

Arterial ulcer
_____

Cellulitis
_____

Dermis
_____

Diabetic ulcer
_____

Grave's disease
_____

Hematoma
_____

Immune system
_____

Venous skin ulcers
_____

Wet-to-dry dressing
_____

You are the triage nurse at a small midwestern hospital. The 68-year-old man in front of you reports that he scraped the side of his leg on the bedpost when he went to the bathroom 2 days ago. He has "doctored" the scrape, and now it is inflamed. All he has done to the area is wash it with antibacterial soap and put an occlusive dressing over it. He states that it is much worse today. The area is red, with minimal gray drainage. You clean the site and ask about his home medications. He hands you a brown paper bag with his medications.

Recent History

You ask about the missing nicotine patch. He tells you that sometimes he forgets and smokes even with the patch on, and when he does, his chest and head hurt. So, most of the time he just keeps the patch off.

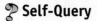

Self-Query

What teaching needs to be done concerning the combination of the nicotine patch and smoking?

_____

_____

Home Medications

Aspirin 81 mg every morning with breakfast orally

Citalopram (Celexa) 20 mg every night before sleep orally

Gemfibrozil (Lopid) 600 mg every morning orally

Levothyroxine sodium (Synthroid) 25 mcg daily every morning orally

Levothyroxine sodium 50 mcg daily every morning orally

Nicotine patch 21 mg placed on the arm every morning (you do not see a patch on either arm)

Tadalafil (Cialis) 2.5 mg 1 hour before sexual activity

Self-Query

Using a drug book or pharmacology text that contains the mechanism of action, unlabeled uses, and pharmacokinetics for medications, answer the following questions. Make answers specific to this scenario.

Do I know why the patient is taking these medications? What do I know about these medications? For each medication, what is the recommended dose, recommended route, and best time of day to give it? Do I know what lab results I need in regard to each medication? Do I know the approved use of each medication? Do I know the most common diseases treated by the listed medications? Are any off-label uses approved for each drug?

Aspirin

_____

_____

Citalopram

_____

_____

Gemfibrozil

_____

_____

Levothyroxine sodium

_____

_____

Nicotine patch

_____

_____

Tadalafil

_____

_____

Do I know the individual's past medical history by looking at the medication list?

_____

_____

Allergies

None

Body Systems

❓ Self-Query

Be prepared to defend your answers.

Can I place each medication under the body system that it commonly affects?

Neurological

_____

Cardiovascular

_____

Hematological

_____

Pulmonary

_____

Gastrointestinal

_____

Nutrition

_____

Genitourinary/renal

_____

Musculoskeletal

_____

Endocrine

_____

Integumentary

_____

Immune

_____

Pain/comfort

_____

Nursing Process

❓ Self-Query

What nursing assessment will I perform regarding each medication? What planning and implementation do I need to do for each medication? How do I evaluate each medication's effectiveness?

Aspirin

_____

_____

Citalopram

_____

_____

Gemfibrozil

_____

_____

Levothyroxine sodium

_____

_____

Nicotine patch

_____

_____

Tadalafil

_____

_____

Are there any geriatric considerations for this individual?

_____

_____

Physician Orders

Cephalexin (Keflex) 500 mg every 12 hours for 7 days
See about the need for tetanus toxoid, and give if needed.

Self-Query

What teaching needs to be done concerning cephalexin?

_____

_____

How will we determine the need for the tetanus? How is tetanus administered?

_____

_____

Synopsis

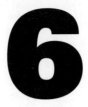

6

Because you can find answers to the self-queries in numerous texts, you will not find the answers to all of them here. However, you will find discussion on the individual case. The scenario relates to circulatory disorders and wound healing; therefore, purposefully look into the medication use and vocabulary as they relate to circulatory patients.

Vocabulary

When reviewing the vocabulary words, you might want to ask several questions: who, what, where, when, why, and how. This should give you a much broader understanding of each word.

Do yourself a favor and do not just give the shortest and simplest answer. Use the following example of the immune system: Instead of answering, "The immune system protects against infections," ask:

What organs are included in the **immune system**? How does it work?

☑ Self-Query: Possible Answers

When defining the remainder of the vocabulary words, ask the following questions:

What is the definition of an **arterial ulcer**? Where are these ulcers located? Who is at risk for arterial ulcers? What commonly causes arterial ulcers? Why would this type of ulcer produce gangrene?

What is **cellulitis**? What is the major cause of cellulitis? What is a medication treatment? Who develops cellulitis?

What is the **dermis**? What is its function? How is it altered by arterial insufficiency? How is it altered by venous insufficiency? How is it altered by diabetes?

What is the pathophysiology behind a **diabetic ulcer**? How is a diabetic ulcer medication induced? Why do they form? Who is at risk for diabetic ulcers? Where are these ulcers located?

What is the pathophysiology of **Grave's disease**? What is the possibility that the person in this scenario has Grave's disease? Who is at risk for developing Grave's disease? How could Grave's disease be medication induced? Which organ is altered in Grave's disease? Why does Grave's disease need to be treated?

What is the pathophysiology of a **hematoma**? Who is at risk for hematomas? Why would certain medications induce the development of a hematoma?

What is the pathophysiology of a **venous skin ulcer**? Who is at risk for venous skin ulcers? Where are these ulcers located? When are these ulcers most likely to develop? Why do venous skin ulcers develop? How are they medication induced?

What is a **wet-to-dry dressing**? Who would most likely benefit from a wet-to-dry dressing? When are they most beneficial? Why would medications be used? Which types of wounds benefit from a wet-to-dry dressing? How are wet-to-dry dressings applied?

Body Systems

☑ Self Query: Possible Answers

Neurological

   Citalopram (Celexa) 20 mg every night before sleep orally

Cardiovascular

   Aspirin 81 mg every morning with breakfast orally
   Gemfibrozil (Lopid) 600 mg every morning orally
   Levothyroxine sodium (Synthroid) 25 mcg daily every morning orally
   Levothyroxine sodium 50 mcg daily every morning orally
   Nicotine patch 21 mg, placed on arm every morning (you do not see a patch on either arm)
   Tadalafil (Cialis) 2.5 mg 1 hour before sexual activity; Tadalafil is not a cardiac medication; however, it is placed here due to the fact that it has cardiac implications (a review of the cardiovascular side effects shows angina/hypotension, for example)

Hematological

   Aspirin 81 mg every morning with breakfast orally

Pulmonary

   Nicotine patch 21 mg placed on arm every morning (you do not see any patch on either arm)
   Tadalafil 2.5 mg 1 hour before sexual activity (review this medication to see treatment research on pulmonary artery hypertension)

Gastrointestinal

   Aspirin 81 mg every morning with breakfast orally (may cause GI bleed)
   Gemfibrozil 600 mg every morning orally

Genitourinary/renal

   Tadalafil 2.5 mg 1 hour before sexual activity

Musculoskeletal

   Gemfibrozil 600 mg every morning orally (may have a detrimental effect on muscles, causing myopathy)

Endocrine

   Levothyroxine sodium 25 mcg daily every morning orally
   Levothyroxine sodium 50 mcg daily every morning orally

Integumentary

   None

Immune

   Tetanus—A person's immunity tends to decline with time, so booster doses are recommended at least every 10 years. However, there is new research on this.

Pain/comfort

   The patient did not identify any pain meds (prescription or over the counter). However, do not assume that he does not take something. Ask!

Aspirin 81 mg every morning with breakfast orally (there are numerous uses for aspirin; at this dose, it is usually used as an antiplatelet)

Citalopram 20 mg every night before sleep orally (SSRI), used to relieve the discomfort associated with depression/insomnia

The medications are not classified as pain medications, but they are given to decrease the pain and discomfort of certain disease processes.

Levothyroxine sodium 25 mcg daily every morning orally

Levothyroxine sodium 50 mcg daily every morning orally

There are varying degrees of hypothyroidism and other thyroid problems, so the proper dosage of levothyroxine sodium will vary from person to person. The recommended dose is based on age, medical conditions, and the results of certain blood tests. Typically, most adults are prescribed between 100 mcg and 125 mcg per day. Some patients need more; some need less.

Tadalafil 2.5 mg 1 hour before sexual activity

Nursing Process

☑ Self-Query: Possible Answers

Regardless of whether we as healthcare providers address it, sexuality is a serious issue with some male patients and their partners. The patient was diagnosed with cellulitis and prescribed Keflex 500 mg orally daily for 7 days. He was scheduled to return to the physician's office in 10 days to assess the wound. He was also administered a tetanus booster.

Teaching: The patient was informed that the injection site of the tetanus booster may be tender to the touch.

Case Study Inquiry

7

Vocabulary

✌ Self-Query

Before attempting to work the case study, define each of the vocabulary words. Although the words may have several subheadings, it will give you a place to begin your inquiry.

Absolute neutrophil count

_____

Alopecia

_____

CA-125

_____

Chemotherapy

_____

Colon cancer

_____

Colostomy

_____

Hand and foot syndrome

_____

Nadir

_____

Neuropathy

_____

Neutrophils

_____

Osteoporosis

_____

Pathologic fracture

_____

Radiation therapy

_____

Tumor markers

_____

You are working on the oncology unit. The patient is a 26-year-old woman who was a direct admit from her oncologist's office after the nurse reported that her white blood cell count was 1200/mm³. You are to assess the patient and review her medications.

Recent History

The patient's husband is at her bedside and answers questions. In the past month, she has recovered from placement of a colostomy due to metastatic ovarian cancer. Her lower right leg has been placed in a cast because of a pathologic fracture. She was at the oncologist for a scheduled round of chemotherapy. She tells you that she is on the following medications for her cancer therapy:

Epoetin alfa (Procrit)

Paclitaxel (Taxol) IV + carboplatin (Paraplatin)

Prednisone orally

Self-Query

What do I know about these medications? For each medication, what is the recommended dose, recommended route, and best time of day to give it? Are these the recommended medications for her type of cancer? Do I know what lab results I need in regard to each medication? Even though I am not giving the medications, what assessment should be completed regarding them?

Epoetin

_____

_____

Paclitaxel IV + carboplatin

_____

_____

Prednisone orally

_____

_____

Do I know how chemotherapy works?

_____

_____

Home Medications

Calcium citrate (Citracal) 2 tabs 3 times a day

Cephalexin (Keflex) 500 mg 3 times a day

Docusate/sennosides (Senokot-S) 2 tabs every 8 hours

Ferrous sulfate 325 mg orally every 6 hours

Furosemide (Lasix) 40 mg daily orally

Gabapentin (Neurontin) 600 mg orally every 8 hours

Granisetron (Kytril) 2 mg daily (2 teaspoons once daily)

Morphine sulfate controlled-release tablets (MS Contin) 30 mg orally every 12 hours

Morphine (MSIR) 10 mg orally as needed for breakthrough pain

Paroxetine (Paxil) 20 mg orally at bedtime and 10 mg every morning

Potassium chloride 20 mEq daily orally

🔑 Self-Query

Using a drug book or pharmacology text that contains the mechanism of action, unlabeled uses, and pharmacokinetics for medications, answer the following questions. Make answers specific to this scenario.

What do I know about these medications? Do I know the recommended dose of, the recommended route for, and the best time of day to give these medications? Do I know what lab results I need regarding each medication? Do I know the approved use of each medication? Do I know the most common diseases treated by the listed medications? Are any off-label uses approved for each drug?

Calcium citrate

_____

_____

Cephalexin

_____

_____

Docusate/sennosides

_____

_____

Ferrous sulfate

_____

_____

Furosemide

_____

_____

Gabapentin

_____

_____

Granisetron

_____

_____

Morphine sulfate controlled-release tablets

_____

_____

Morphine

_____

_____

Paroxetine

_____

_____

Potassium chloride

_____

_____

Do I know the individual's possible past medical history by looking at the medications?

_____

_____

What is the connection between ferrous sulfate and epoetin alfa?

_____

_____

Why Senokot-S and not plain Senokot? What is the "S" in Senokot-S?

_____

_____

Why granisetron and not promethazine (Phenergan) or prochlorperzine (Compazine)?

_____

_____

What other serotonin receptor antagonist would be appropriate for nausea?

_____

_____

Does the individual have a past medical history other than the cancer?

_____

_____

Allergies

No known drug allergies

Body Systems

Self-Query

Be prepared to defend your answers.

Can I place each medication under the body system which it commonly affects?
Neurological

_____

Cardiovascular

_____

Hematological

_____

Pulmonary

_____

Gastrointestinal

_____

Nutrition

_____

Genitourinary/renal

_____

Musculoskeletal

_____

Endocrine

_____

Integumentary

_____

Immune

_____

Pain/comfort

_____

Mechanism of Action

？ Self-Query

Does the individual's medical history have an effect on the pharmacokinetics of the drug?

_____

_____

What contraindications do I need to address regarding the medications and this individual's health history?

_____

_____

Nursing Process

？ Self-Query

What nursing assessment will I perform regarding each medication? What planning and implementation do I need for each medication? How do I evaluate each medication's effectiveness?

Calcium citrate

_____

_____

Cephalexin

_____

_____

Docusate/sennosides

_____

_____

Epoetin alfa

_____

_____

Ferrous sulfate

_____

_____

Furosemide

_____

_____

Gabapentin

_____

_____

Granisetron

_____

_____

Morphine sulfate controlled-release tablets

_____

_____

Morphine

_____

_____

Paclitaxel IV + carboplatin

_____

_____

Paroxetine

_____

_____

Potassium chloride

_____

_____

Prednisone orally

_____

_____

Physical Assessment Findings
Neurological Assessment

Opens eyes to verbal stimuli, follows verbal commands, minimal verbal response.
Weak grips, plantar dorsiflexion and extension weak on affected extremity.

Cardiac Assessment

Heart sounds S_1S_2 irregular; cardiac monitor reveals sinus rhythm with frequent premature ventricular beats, distant heart sounds, radial pulses 1+ to right foot dorsalis pedis; 2+ to left dorsalis pedis, with noted trace edema to hands and feet. Blood pressure 102/50, skin warm and dry, capillary refill < 3 seconds K+ −3.0.

Pulmonary Assessment

Respiratory rate 16, no respiratory distress, skin warm and dry, pale mucous membranes.

Gastrointestinal Assessment

Soft, nondistended abdomen, bowel sounds hypoactive in all quadrants, colostomy stoma pink. Semiformed stool to bag. Noted minimal stomatitis. The patient states that she had nausea this morning before the office visit. Small, white patches noted in oral cavity. The patient states that she is thirsty and has had two bouts of nausea. The patient weighs 110 pounds and is 5′7″ tall.

Genitourinary Assessment

Assisted to void upon admission, noted 200 mL dark yellow urine, no burning upon urination.

Musculoskeletal Assessment

Moves all extremities; cast noted to lower right extremity; no odor; unable to walk because of weakness and cast.

Endocrine Assessment

No exophthalmos, no slow-healing wounds, no goiter; noted history of diabetes.

Integumentary Assessment

Warm to touch, patches of dry skin, noted alopecia, noted hyperpigmentation to nail beds and gums.

Immune Assessment

Lab results: platelets—10,000/mm^3; WBC—1200/mm^3; neutrophils % 34 ANC=408.

Pain/Comfort Assessment

Reports pain level of 8 on a 1–10 scale.

Physician Orders

Stop cephalexin

Neutropenic precautions

Complete blood count/platelet count

Serum creatinine

Fluconazole (Diflucan) 200 mg IV daily

Normal saline 150 mL/hr

Potassium 40 mEq IV

Filgrastim (Neupogen) 5 mcg/kg/day, IV infusion daily until the ANC has reached 1,000/m^3.

Infuse 2 units of fresh frozen plasma

What classification are these medications? Why is each medication usually given? How is it usually given? Why was each medication ordered for this patient?

Fluconazole

_____

_____

Filgrastim

_____

_____

Potassium

_____

_____

Nursing Process

Self-Query

What nursing assessment will I perform regarding each medication? What planning and implementation do I need to conduct for each medication? How do I evaluate each medication's effectiveness?

Fluconazole

_____

_____

Filgrastim

_____

_____

Potassium

_____

_____

Is there a need to replace the cephalexin?

_____

What do I think happened to this individual and why? (Be specific.)

_____

_____

_____

Synopsis

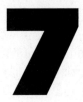

7

Because you can find answers to the self-queries in numerous texts, you will not find the answers to all of them here. However, you will find discussion of the individual case. The scenario relates to complications of chemotherapy; therefore, purposefully look into the medication use and vocabulary as they relate to oncology patients.

Vocabulary

When reviewing the vocabulary words, you might want to ask several questions: who, what, where, when, why, and how. This should give you a much broader understanding of each word.

Do yourself a favor and do not just give the shortest and simplest answer. Use the following example of osteoporosis: Instead of answering, "Osteoporosis is a bone disease that increases the risk of fractures," ask:

What is the pathophysiology of **osteoporosis**? Who is at risk for osteoporosis? Where is it found in the body? Why is it important to treat osteoporosis? How might it be related to chemotherapy, considering the scenario's cancer medications?

☑ Self-Query: Possible Answers

When defining the remainder of the vocabulary words, ask the following questions:

What is the **absolute neutrophil count** (ANC)? Who is affected by a low ANC? How is it calculated? What does it tell us? Why is it important? How might it be related to chemotherapy, considering this scenario's cancer medications?

What is **alopecia**? How might it be related to chemotherapy, considering this scenario's cancer medications? Why is it not usually a permanent condition? What are two medications known to cause alopecia?

What is the **CA-125**? What does the CA stand for? Why would a physician order it? How is it used in finding cancer cells?

What is **chemotherapy**? How does chemotherapy for cancer work? In this scenario, which medications are considered cancer medications? What are two major **side effects** of the scenario's cancer medications?

How is **colon cancer** diagnosed? Who is at risk for colon cancer? What medications are prescribed in the treatment of colon cancer? In this scenario, is the colon cancer primary or metastatic in nature?

What is a **colostomy**? Who might need a colostomy? Why is a colostomy needed? How does the location of the colostomy determine the consistency of the stool?

What is **hand and foot syndrome**? What is the medical term for hand and foot syndrome? How is it treated? How might it be related to chemotherapy, considering this scenario's cancer medications? Is it a permanent condition? What two medications are primarily known to cause hand and foot syndrome? What body system is primarily altered?

What is a **nadir**? How is it related to chemotherapy, considering this scenario's cancer medications? Who has a nadir measured? What system is most affected?

What is **neuropathy**? Who might develop neuropathy? What symptoms might a person report who is developing neuropathy? How might it be related to chemotherapy, considering the scenario's cancer medications?

What is a **neutrophil**? What is the function of the neutrophil? How long do neutrophils live? What are mature neutrophils called? What are immature neutrophils called? How are neutrophils related to the chemotherapy, considering this scenario's cancer medications?

What is a **pathologic fracture**? Who is at risk for these types of fractures? When are these fractures most likely to occur? Where in the skeletal system are these fractures most likely to be found? How might a pathologic fracture relate to chemotherapy, considering the cancer medications in this scenario?

What is **radiation therapy**? Who is a candidate for radiation therapy? How is it used to treat cancer?

What is a **tumor marker**? Why are tumor markers used? How do chemotherapy medications affect tumor markers?

Body Systems

☑ Self-Query: Possible Answers

Neurological

Gabapentin (Neurontin) 600 mg orally every 8 hours

Morphine sulfate controlled-release tablets (MS Contin) 30 mg orally every 12 hours

Morphine (MSIR) 10 mg orally as needed for breakthrough pain

Note that both of the following medications (Granisetron [Kytril] and paroxetine [Paxil]) are related to serotonin, a neurotransmitter:

Granisetron 2 mg daily (2 teaspoons once daily)—granisetron works by blocking the serotonin (5-HT3) receptor. Patients receiving certain cancer treatment medications have the hormone serotonin released by cells in the small intestine. Serotonin then acts on the vagus nerve to trigger nausea and vomiting. Granisetron decreases the effect by blocking serotonin receptors on the vagus nerve, reducing stimulation by serotonin.

Paroxetine 20 mg orally at bedtime and 10 mg every morning—paroxetine is an antidepressant medication known as a selective serotonin reuptake inhibitor (SSRI). Depression and anxiety disorders may be related to certain neurotransmitters. Serotonin is only one neurotransmitter. Serotonin is released from one nerve cell and travels to the next. During the sending and receiving of this neurotransmitter, serotonin is either absorbed or returned to the original sender cell. Paroxetine treats depression and anxiety by keeping serotonin from being reabsorbed into the sender nerve cell.

Cardiovascular

Ferrous sulfate 325 mg orally every 6 hours

Furosemide (Lasix) 40 mg daily orally

Paclitaxel (Taxol) IV + carboplatin (Paraplatin) can alter the heart's function.

Potassium chloride 20 mEq daily orally

In chemo:

Epoetin alfa (Procrit)

Paclitaxel IV + carboplatin

Prednisone orally

Hematological

Calcium citrate (Citracal) 2 tabs 3 times a day

Cephalexin (Keflex) 500 mg 3 times a day (stopped on admission to the hospital)

Ferrous sulfate 325 mg orally every 6 hours

Filgrastim (Neupogen) 5 mcg/kg/day IV (added at the hospital)

Fluconazole (Diflucan) 200 mg IV daily (added at the hospital)

Furosemide 40 mg daily orally

Potassium chloride 20 mEq daily orally

Reviewing the physical assessment, we see a severely compromised bone marrow. Bone marrow suppression is a major dose-limiting toxicity; this is the reason for neutropenic precautions. Paclitaxel and carboplatin can affect the hematological and cardiovascular system.

In chemo:

Epoetin alfa

Paclitaxel IV + carboplatin

Prednisone orally

Pulmonary

Furosemide 40 mg daily orally

Paclitaxel IV + carboplatin can alter the pulmonary, heart, and hematological systems.

In chemo:

Epoetin alfa

Paclitaxel IV + carboplatin

Prednisone orally

Gastrointestinal

Calcium citrate 2 tabs 3 times a day

Docusate/sennosides (Senokot-S) 2 tabs every 8 hours

Ferrous sulfate 325 mg orally every 6 hours

Granisetron 2 mg daily (2 teaspoons once daily)

The following chemo medications have detrimental effects on the GI system (which begins in the mouth):

Epoetin alfa

Paclitaxel IV + carboplatin

Prednisone orally

Genitourinary/renal

Furosemide 40 mg daily orally

Potassium chloride 20 mEq daily orally

Musculoskeletal

Calcium citrate 2 tabs 3 times a day

Gabapentin 600 mg orally every 8 hours

Morphine 10 mg orally as needed for breakthrough pain

Morphine sulfate controlled-release tablets 30 mg orally every 12 hours

Endocrine

None specific to this system.

Integumentary

Cephalexin 500 mg 3 times a day (stopped on admission to the hospital)

Fluconazole 200 mg IV daily (added at the hospital)

Immune

Ferrous sulfate 325 mg orally every 6 hours

Filgrastim 5 mcg/kg/day IV (added at the hospital)

Fluconazole 200 mg IV daily (added at the hospital)

In chemo:

    Epoetin alfa

    Paclitaxel IV + carboplatin

    Prednisone orally

Pain/comfort

Docusate/sennosides 2 tabs every 8 hours

Filgrastim 5 mcg/kg/day IV (added at hospital)

Fluconazole 200 mg IV daily (added at hospital)

Gabapentin 600 mg orally every 8 hours

Granisetron 2 mg daily (2 teaspoons once daily)

Morphine 10 mg orally as needed for breakthrough pain

Morphine sulfate controlled-release tablets 30 mg orally every 12 hours

Paroxetine 20 mg orally at bedtime and 10 mg every morning

Nursing Process

☑ Self-Query: Possible Answers

The patient's scheduled treatment of chemotherapy was postponed because of her ANC. She was dehydrated. Epoetin alfa cannot work efficiently if the patient's iron stores are deficient. This includes transferrin saturation (serum iron divided by iron-binding capacity) and serum ferritin.

Senokot-S is a laxative that includes a softener. Do your patients a favor and include a softener and a laxative in their prescribed medications if they are taking any opioid.

Antiemetics: Granisetron is a serotonin receptor antagonist. These are the most effective antiemetic medications prescribed for nausea and vomiting induced by paclitaxel + carboplatin.

Promethazine (Phenergan) and prochlorperazine (Compazine) are effective antiemetics. However, they have other side effects that may add to the patient's discomfort. Prednisone can also be used as an antiemetic.

The patient suffered from neutropenia (ANC of 408) as a result of the paclitaxel + carboplatin and the filgrastim administration. The patient also suffered cardiac damage trace edema to hands and feet. Assessment of the oral cavity and presence of white patches revealed candida, thus, the prescription for the fluconazole, an antifungal. Cast placement was the result of a pathological fracture.

As to the question, "Is there a need to replace the cephalexin?" no antibiotic replaced the cephalexin at the insistence of the patient and her husband. Cephalexin can actually cause an adverse reaction, neutropenia, in some patients. It is also known to cause candidiasis. Once it was stopped and the other medications were given as prescribed, the patient recovered as much as possible and continued her therapy.

The cast was removed for further assessment and replaced with a brace.

Different hospitals use various guidelines regarding prevention of and treatment for infections.

Medications are prescribed with regard to renal and hepatic function. This is one of the reasons for the serum creatinine and complete blood count (CBC).

The patient was afebrile, and there was no evidence of any other infection besides the oral candida. All antifungal and antibiotic treatment should be prescribed with regard to the cultures and susceptibility of the organism and the host's renal and hepatic function, particularly those patients receiving medications that alter the function of so many systems.

Always assess for myelosuppression and immunocompromise in individuals receiving chemotherapy medications.

Case Study Inquiry

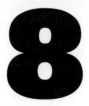

Vocabulary

Self-Query

Before attempting to work the case study, define each of the vocabulary words. Although the words may have several subheadings, it will give you a place to begin your inquiry.

Anemia

_____

Antianginal

_____

Benign prostate hypertrophy

_____

Calcium channel blocker

_____

Cholesterol

_____

Dyspnea

_____

Hyperlipidemia

_____

Medication reconciliation

_____

Orthopnea

_____

Platelet

_____

Water pill

_____

Your 85-year-old patient is being discharged home after recovering from an exacerbation of congestive heart failure. He asks you to review his home medications with him and his daughter.

Recent History

The patient stated that he began coughing up "thick pink sputum." He had not felt well for several days and noticed that his shoes and socks were a little tight. He stated that he took an extra "water pill" and called his daughter. When she arrived, he was having difficulty breathing. She brought him to the emergency room. That was a week ago. He has been in critical care, and now, after a few days on the step-down unit, he is being discharged. His family wants to help keep a closer eye on him and his medicines.

Home Medications

Amlodipine (Norvasc) 10 mg daily orally

Aspirin and dipyridamole (Aggrenox) 1 capsule twice a day orally

Atenolol (Tenormin) 50 mg daily orally

Clonidine (Catapres) 0.1 mg daily orally

Docusate (Colace) 1 cap at bedtime

Furosemide (Lasix) 80 mg every morning orally

Hydrocodone 10/acetaminophen 325 (Vicodin) 1 tab every 6 hours as needed for pain

Isosorbide (Imdur) 60 mg every morning orally

Potassium chloride 20 mEq daily orally

Ranitidine (Zantac) 150 mg daily orally

Self-Query

Using a drug book or pharmacology text that contains the mechanism of action, unlabeled uses, and pharmacokinetics for medications, answer the following questions. Make answers specific to this scenario.

What do I know about these medications? Do I know the recommended dose of, the recommended route for, and the best time of day to give these medications? Do I know what lab results I need regarding each medication? Do I know the approved use of each medication? Do I know the most common diseases treated by the listed medications? Are any off-label uses approved for each drug?

Amlodipine

_____

_____

Aspirin and dipyridamole

_____

_____

Atenolol

_____

_____

Clonidine

_____

_____

Docusate

_____

_____

Furosemide

_____

_____

Hydrocodone 10/acetaminophen 325

_____

_____

Isosorbide

_____

_____

Potassium chloride

_____

_____

Ranitidine

_____

_____

Do I know the individual's past medical history by looking at the medications?

_____

_____

Allergies

Fluconazole (Diflucan)

Morphine sulfate extended release (Kadian)

Self-Query

Do I know why each of these medications is used? Do I know the signs and symptoms of an adverse reaction to each of these medications?

Fluconazole

_____

_____

Morphine sulfate extended release

_____

_____

Do I know what other drugs this individual may be allergic to, given his allergy to morphine sulfate extended release?

_____

_____

Body Systems

? **Self-Query**

Be prepared to defend your answers.

Can I place each medication under the body system that it commonly affects?

Neurological

_____

Cardiovascular

_____

Hematological

_____

Pulmonary

_____

Gastrointestinal

_____

Nutrition

_____

Genitourinary/renal

_____

Musculoskeletal

_____

Endocrine

_____

Integumentary

_____

Immune

_____

Pain/comfort

_____

Patient Request

The 85-year-old patient asks you to write a description of his medications so he can keep it next to them in his kitchen.

? **Self-Query**

What will you teach him, and what will you write?

Nursing Process

? **Self-Query**

What nursing assessment should be performed regarding each medication? What planning and implementation should the patient and family do in regard to each medication? How do the patient and family evaluate each medication's effectiveness?

Discuss the findings with the class.

Amlodipine

_____

_____

Aspirin and dipyridamole

_____

_____

Atenolol

_____

_____

Clonidine

_____

_____

Docusate

_____

_____

Furosemide

_____

_____

Hydrocodone 10/acetaminophen 325

_____

_____

Isosorbide

_____

_____

Potassium chloride

_____

_____

Ranitidine

_____

_____

Synopsis

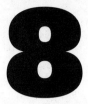

Because you can find answers to the self-queries in numerous texts, you will not find the answers to all of them here. However, you will find discussion of the individual case. The scenario relates to heart failure; therefore, purposefully look into the medication use and vocabulary as they relate to heart failure patients.

Vocabulary

When reviewing the vocabulary words, you might want to ask several questions: who, what, where, when, why, and how. This should give you a much broader understanding of each word.

Do yourself a favor and do not just give the shortest and simplest answer. Use the following example for medication reconciliation: Instead of answering, "The medication reconciliation compares all of a patient's medication orders with all the medications that the patient has been taking," ask:

Why perform a **medication reconciliation**, and when is it performed? What are medication reconciliations? Who performs medication reconciliations? Where are they done? How are they done?

☑ Self-Query: Possible Answers

When defining the remainder of the vocabulary words, ask the following questions:

What is the definition of **anemia**? Who develops anemia? Why is anemia considered a symptom? Might this patient suffer from anemia even though he has no medications suggesting this? Might there be a connection between some of his medications and the anemia? Explain. How could his anemia also be related to age?

What is angina? Who develops angina? What is an **antianginal** medication? How do we know that this man may have had angina in the past?

Where is the prostate located? What age group most often develops problems? Why would **benign prostate hypertrophy (BPH)** be considered age related? How can medications help this problem? What body system is altered?

What do **calcium channel blockers (CCBs)** block? Where is the calcium channel located? How do these medications relate to hypertension? Who is usually prescribed a CCB?

What is **cholesterol**? How is it related to lipids? What role does cholesterol play in the body? What medication(s) is the patient taking that will affect his cholesterol?

What is **dyspnea**? What medication(s) is the patient taking that will affect dyspnea? How is his dyspnea related to lack of medication?

What role do lipids play in the body? What is the pathophysiology of **hyperlipidemia**? Who is at risk for hyperlipidemia? What commonly causes hyperlipidemia? Why is it important to receive medication treatment for hyperlipidemia?

What is **orthopnea**? What medication(s) is the patient taking that will affect orthopnea? How is orthopnea related to disease? How is orthopnea indicative of heart disease? Why is orthopnea more indicative of heart disease than dyspnea?

What medication(s) is the patient taking that will affect his **platelets**? How long does a platelet live? Why are platelets needed?

In this scenario, which medication is the patient calling his "**water pill**"?

Body Systems

☑ Self-Query: Possible Answers

Neurological

Any of these medications can be detrimental neurologically in the geriatric individual.
Hydrocodone 10/acetaminophen 325 (Vicodin) 1 tab every 6 hours as needed for pain

Cardiovascular

Amlodipine (Norvasc) 10 mg daily orally
Aspirin and dipyridamole (Aggrenox) 1 capsule twice a day orally
Potassium chloride 20 mEq daily orally
Atenolol (Tenormin) 50 mg daily orally
Clonidine (Catapres) 0.1 mg daily orally
Furosemide (Lasix) 80 mg every morning orally
Isosorbide (Imdur) 60 mg every morning orally

Hematological

Potassium chloride 20 mEq daily orally

Pulmonary

Any of these medications can be detrimental to the pulmonary system in the geriatric individual.

Gastrointestinal

Any of these medications can be detrimental to the GI system in the geriatric individual.
Ranitidine (Zantac) 150 mg daily orally
Docusate (Colace) 1 cap at bedtime

Nutrition

Be aware that this geriatric individual will most likely have nutritional deficits, which will alter protein binding and the levels of the medications available in the system.

Genitourinary/renal

Be aware that this geriatric individual will most likely have some age-related decreased renal function. This will alter excretion and the levels of the medications remaining in the system.
Potassium chloride 20 mEq daily orally
Furosemide 80 mg every morning orally

Musculoskeletal

Any of these medications can be detrimental in the geriatric individual, particularly the cardiovascular medications, which may lead to hypotension and cause the patient to lose balance.

Integumentary

Any of these medications can be detrimental to the geriatric individual's skin.

Immune

> Any of these medications can be detrimental to the geriatric individual. Note that the immunity of the geriatric individual is decreased.

Pain/comfort

> Consider that all the medications are to relieve symptoms that cause pain and discomfort.
> Hydrocodone 10/acetaminophen 325 1 tab every 6 hours as needed for pain
> Amlodipine 10 mg daily orally
> Aspirin and dipyridamole 1 capsule twice a day orally
> Potassium chloride 20 mEq daily orally
> Atenolol 50 mg daily orally
> Clonidine 0.1 mg daily orally
> Furosemide 80 mg every morning orally
> Isosorbide 60 mg every morning orally
> Hydrocodone 10/acetaminophen 325 1 tab every 6 hours as needed for pain
> Ranitidine 150 mg daily orally
> Ducosate 1 cap at bedtime

Nursing Process

☑ Self-Query: Possible Answers

The patient was diagnosed with pulmonary edema, and the medications in critical care were not addressed.

Fluconazole (Diflucan) had been prescribed in the past for a fungal eye infection. It was not an allergy; however, he has a long history of alcohol consumption. Fluconazole is not to be taken when ethanol (ETOH) is consumed.

Kadian is sustained-release morphine and can be administered only once a day. It was not a true allergy; the patient was afraid that he would become addicted after he discovered that Kadian is morphine. It was prescribed because he had pain related to vascular disease and osteoarthritis. He had no objection to the hydrocodone 10/acetaminophen 325.

Case Study Inquiry

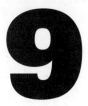

Vocabulary

🔖 Self-Query

Before attempting to work the case study, define the vocabulary words. Although the words may have several subheadings, it will give you a place to begin your inquiry.

Bone demineralization
___

Cystitis
___

Osteoporosis
___

Spasticity
___

Stress incontinence
___

Urinary tract infection
___

Your 75-year-old female patient is in the clinic today with reports of burning upon urination. Before the nurse practitioner sees her, you are reviewing her medications. She hands you the list she carries with her.

Home Medications

Alendronate (Fosamax) 70 mg every morning 30 minutes before breakfast
Alprazolam (Xanax) 0.25 mg every morning with other medications
Aspirin (ASA) 81 mg daily at 10 a.m.
Baclofen 10 mg every morning upon waking
Furosemide (Lasix) 40 mg 2 times a day (10 a.m. and 6 p.m.)
Glycerin suppository, 1 every morning as needed
Metoprolol tartrate (Lopressor) 12.5 mg twice a day (10 a.m. and 6 p.m.)
Multivitamin 1 tab every morning with other medications
Omega-3 one 1000-mg tab every morning with breakfast
Potassium chloride 20 mEq taken with the furosemide
Solifenacin succinate (VESIcare) 10 mg every morning with the furosemide

🔖 Self-Query

Using a drug book or pharmacology text that contains the mechanism of action, unlabeled uses, and pharmacokinetics for medications, answer the following questions. Make answers specific to this scenario.

What do I know about these medications? Do I know the recommended dose of, the recommended route for, and the best time of day to give these medications? Do I know what lab results I need regarding each medication? Do I know the approved use of each medication? Do I know the most common diseases treated by the listed medications? Are any off-label uses approved for each drug?

Alendronate

_____

_____

Alprazolam

_____

_____

Aspirin

_____

_____

Baclofen

_____

_____

Furosemide

_____

_____

Glycerin suppository

_____

_____

Metoprolol tartrate

_____

_____

Multivitamin

_____

_____

Omega-3

_____

_____

Potassium chloride

_____

_____

Solifenacin succinate

_____

_____

Do I know the individual's past medical history by looking at the medication list?

_____

_____

Allergies

Meperidine (Demerol)

Self-Query

Do I know why meperidine is used? Do I know the signs and symptoms of an adverse reaction to meperidine?

_____

_____

What are the contraindications for meperidine in this age group?

_____

Body Systems

Self-Query

Be prepared to defend your answers.

Can I place each medication under the body system that it commonly affects?

Neurological

_____

Cardiovascular

_____

Hematological

_____

Pulmonary

_____

Gastrointestinal

_____

Nutrition

_____

Genitourinary/renal

_____

Musculoskeletal

_____

Endocrine

_____

Integumentary

_____

Immune

_____

Pain/comfort

_____

Mechanism of Action

Self-Query

Does the individual's medical history have an effect on the pharmacokinetics of each drug?

_____

_____

What contraindications do I need to address regarding the medications and medical history?

_____

_____

Nursing Process

? Self-Query

What nursing assessment will I perform regarding each medication? What planning and implementation do I need to do in regard to each medication? How do I evaluate each medication's effectiveness?

Alendronate

_____

_____

Alprazolam

_____

_____

Aspirin

_____

_____

Baclofen

_____

_____

Furosemide

_____

_____

Glycerin suppository

_____

_____

Metoprolol tartrate

_____

_____

Multivitamin

_____

_____

Omega-3

_____

_____

Potassium chloride

_____

_____

Solifenacin succinate

_____

_____

Do I need to be concerned about geriatric considerations for this individual?

_____

Synopsis

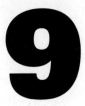

Because you can find answers to the self-queries in numerous texts, you will not find the answers to all of them here. However, you will find discussion of the individual case. The scenario relates to the geriatric individual diagnosed with muscle spasms and spasticity; therefore, purposefully look into the medication use and vocabulary as they relate to these issues.

Vocabulary

When reviewing the vocabulary words, you might want to ask several questions: who, what, where, when, why, and how. This should give you a much broader understanding of each word.

Do yourself a favor and do not just give the shortest and simplest answer. Use the following example of cystitis: Instead of answering, "Cystitis is an inflammation of the urinary bladder," ask:

What is the pathophysiology of **cystitis**? Who is at risk for cystitis? What commonly causes cystitis? How is it medication induced?

☑ Self-Query: Possible Answers

When defining the remainder of the vocabulary words, ask the following questions:

What is the pathophysiology of **bone demineralization**? What is bone demineralization? Why is it a symptom of greater problems? Why is it sometimes treatment induced? Who is at risk for bone demineralization? What medications can result in bone demineralization?

What is **osteoporosis**? What medication(s) is this individual taking that will alter osteoporosis? How is the patient's osteoporosis in the scenario medication related? Who is at risk for osteoporosis?

What is **spasticity**? What is the pathophysiology of spasticity? Who is at risk for spasticity? What diseases commonly cause spasticity? How is it medication/disease induced?

What is **stress incontinence**? What is the pathophysiology of stress incontinence? Who is at risk for stress incontinence? How is it medication/disease induced?

What is a **urinary tract infection (UTI)**? Who is at risk for a UTI? How is a UTI related to cystitis?

Body Systems

☑ Self Query: Possible Answers

Neurological

> Any of these medications can be detrimental neurologically in the geriatric individual.
> Alprazolam (Xanax) 0.25 mg every morning with other medications
> Baclofen 10 mg every morning upon waking up
> Solifenacin succinate (VESIcare) 10 mg every morning with furosemide (Lasix)

Cardiovascular

Aspirin (ASA) 81 mg daily at 10 a.m.
Furosemide 40 mg twice a day (10 a.m. and 6 p.m.)
Metoprolol tartrate (Lopressor) 12.5 mg twice a day (10 a.m. and 6 p.m.)
Potassium chloride 20 mEq taken with the furosemide

Hematological

Aspirin 81 mg daily at 10 a.m.
Furosemide 40 mg twice a day (10 a.m. and 6 p.m.)
Multivitamin 1 tab every morning with other medications
Omega 3 one 1000-mg tab every morning with breakfast
Potassium chloride 20 mEq taken with the furosemide

Pulmonary

Although no specific medications are related to this system, be aware that any medication may alter this system, particularly in the geriatric individual.

Gastrointestinal

Any of these medications can be detrimental to the GI system in the geriatric individual.
Glycerin suppository, 1 every morning as needed

Nutrition

Be aware that this geriatric individual will most likely have nutritional deficits. This will alter protein binding and the levels of the medications available in the system.
Multivitamin 1 tab every morning with other medications
Omega 3 one 1000-mg tab every morning with breakfast

Genitourinary/renal

Be aware that this geriatric individual will most likely have some age-related decreased renal function. This will alter excretion and the levels of the medications remaining in the system.
Furosemide 40 mg twice a day (10 a.m. and 6 p.m.)
Solifenacin succinate 10 mg every morning with the furosemide

Musculoskeletal

Alendronate (Fosamax) 70 mg every morning 30 minutes before breakfast
Baclofen 10 mg every morning upon waking up
Solifenacin succinate 10 mg every morning with the furosemide

Endocrine

Although no specific medications are related to this system, be aware that any medication may alter this system, particularly in the geriatric individual.

Integumentary

Although no specific medications are related to this system, be aware that any medication may alter this system, particularly in the geriatric individual.

Immune

Although no specific medications are related to this system, be aware that any medication may alter this system, particularly in the geriatric individual.

Pain/comfort

 Although there are no "pain meds" on her list, the patient probably takes an OTC pain medication.
   Consider that all the medications are to relieve symptoms that cause pain and discomfort.
 Alendronate 70 mg every morning 30 minutes before breakfast
 Alprazolam 0.25 mg every morning with other medications
 Aspirin 81 mg daily at 10 a.m.
 Baclofen 10 mg every morning upon waking up
 Furosemide 40 mg twice a day (10 a.m. and 6 p.m.)
 Glycerin suppository, 1 every morning as needed
 Metoprolol tartrate 12.5 mg twice a day (10 a.m. and 6 p.m.)
 Multivitamin 1 tab every morning with other medications
 Omega 3 one 1000-mg tab every morning with breakfast
 Potassium chloride 20 mEq taken with the furosemide
 Solifenacin succinate 10 mg every morning with the furosemide

Nursing Process

☑ Self-Query: Possible Answers

The patient was diagnosed with a urinary tract infection, which is common in postmenopausal women with urinary incontinence. She has a history of a spinal cord injury that was repaired 25 years ago; with age, her spinal column has further deteriorated, and she has developed hyperactive reflexes.

She has a medical history of urge incontinence, which leads to an incomplete emptying of the bladder. This can be a risk factor for UTIs. Her reaction to meperidine (Demerol) included urinary retention, hives, and severe itching. For the itching, she stated that she took Benadryl (an anticholinergic medication), which also caused urinary retention.

Case Study Inquiry

10

Vocabulary

Self-Query

Before attempting to work the case study, define each of the vocabulary words. Although the words may have several subheadings, it will give you a place to begin your inquiry.

Crohn's disease

_____

Fistula

_____

Ileostomy

_____

Ileum

_____

Intestinal obstruction

_____

Koch pouch

_____

Single-barrel stoma

_____

Ulcerative colitis

_____

Your 59-year-old male patient is in the clinic today reporting that he thinks something is wrong with his week-old ileostomy. He also reports burning during urination. Before the nurse practitioner sees the patient, you review his medications. He does not have a list of medications, so you review his chart and then review his medications with him.

Home Medications

Atropine 0.3 mg every 4–6 hours as needed

Chlordiazepoxide (Librium) 5 mg every 8 hours

Cholestyramine (Questran) 4 mg every morning

Desvenlafaxine (Pristiq) 50 mg 1 tab every morning

Ibuprofen (Motrin) 800 mg as needed for pain

Potassium chloride 10 mEq 1 tab every morning

Sildenafil (Viagra) 25 mg 1 hour before sexual activity

Using a drug book or pharmacology text that contains the mechanism of action, unlabeled uses, and pharmacokinetics for medications, answer the following questions. Make answers specific to this scenario.

What do I know about these medications? Do I know the recommended dose of, the recommended route for, and the best time of day to give these medications? Do I know what lab results I need regarding each medication? Do I know the approved use of each medication? Do I know the most common diseases treated by the listed medications? Are any off-label uses approved for each drug?

Atropine

_____

_____

Chlordiazepoxide

_____

_____

Cholestyramine

_____

_____

Desvenlafaxine

_____

_____

Ibuprofen

_____

_____

Potassium chloride

_____

_____

Sildenafil

_____

_____

Do I know the individual's possible past medical history by looking at the medications?

_____

_____

Allergies

Gentamicin

Phenobarbital

? Self-Query

Do I know why each medication was previously used? Do I know the signs and symptoms of an adverse reaction to each medication? Do I know the classification of each medication?

Gentamicin

_____

_____

Phenobarbital

_____

_____

What drug is the patient taking that possibly replaced the phenobarbital?

_____

Body Systems

Self-Query

Be prepared to defend your answers.

Can I place each medication under the body system that it commonly affects?

Neurological

_____

Cardiovascular

_____

Hematological

_____

Pulmonary

_____

Gastrointestinal

_____

Nutrition

_____

Genitourinary/renal

_____

Musculoskeletal

_____

Endocrine

_____

Integumentary

_____

Immune

_____

Pain/comfort

_____

Mechanism of Action

Self-Query

Does the individual's medical history have an effect on the pharmacokinetics of each drug?

_____

_____

What contraindications do I need to address regarding the medications and medical history?

_____

_____

Nursing Process

Self-Query

What nursing assessment will I perform regarding each medication? What planning and implementation do I need to do in regard to each medication? How do I evaluate each medication's effectiveness?

Atropine

_____

_____

Chlordiazepoxide

_____

_____

Cholestyramine

_____

_____

Desvenlafaxine

_____

_____

Ibuprofen

_____

_____

Potassium chloride

_____

_____

Sildenafil

_____

_____

Physician Orders

Ciprofloxacin (Cipro) 500 mg 1 pill daily for 10 days, pending results of urine culture

Synopsis

10

Because you can find answers to the self-queries in numerous texts, you will not find the answers to all of them here. However, you will find discussion of the individual cases. The scenario relates to gastrointestinal disorders and ileostomies; therefore, purposefully look into the medication use and vocabulary as they relate to gastrointestinal disorders and ileostomies.

Vocabulary

When reviewing the vocabulary words, you might want to ask several questions: who, what, where, when, why, and how. This should give you a much broader understanding of each word.

Do yourself a favor and do not just give the shortest and simplest answer. The following questions are to be used as a guide. Use the example of ileostomy: Instead of answering, "The ileostomy is a surgically created opening in the abdominal wall through which fecal material can pass," ask:

Why is an **ileostomy** done? Where is an ileostomy placed? Who is at risk for needing an ileostomy? How is the placement determined?

☑ Self-Query: Possible Answers

When defining the remainder of the vocabulary words, ask the following questions:

What is the pathophysiology of **Crohn's disease**? List three types of people who are at risk for Crohn's. What medications is the man in the scenario receiving that may be used for Crohn's? Is Crohn's disease medication induced? What body system is altered?

What is a **fistula** in the gastrointestinal tract? Is a fistula medication or disease related?

Where is the **ileum** located?

What is an **intestinal obstruction**? Where can the intestinal obstruction be located? Is the person diagnosed with Crohn's disease or UC at risk for an intestinal obstruction?

What is a **Koch pouch**? Where is the pouch located? Is the person diagnosed with Crohn's disease a candidate for the pouch?

What is a **single-barrel stoma**? Where can the stoma be located? Is the person diagnosed with Crohn's disease or UC a candidate for the single-barrel stoma?

What is the pathophysiology of **ulcerative colitis (UC)**? List three types of people who are at risk for UC. What medications is the man in the scenario receiving that may be used for UC? Is UC medication induced? What body system is altered?

Body Systems

☑ Self-Query: Possible Answers

Neurological

> Desvenlafaxine (Pristiq) 50 mg 1 tab every morning (a serotonin-norepinephrine reuptake inhibitor approved to treat adult patients with major depressive disorder)

Chlordiazepoxide (Librium) 5 mg every 8 hours
Ibuprofen (Motrin) 800 mg as needed for pain
Allergies: Phenobarbital (PB), an anticonvulsant, was tried along with other medications to decrease the symptoms of Crohn's disease. The patient became severely drowsy and refused to take the medication.

Cardiovascular

Atropine 0.3 mg every 4–6 hours as needed
Has a cardiovascular effect, but was not given for the heart.
Its primary effect is in the GI system for this patient.
Be aware that there is no way to avoid an effect on the cardiac system.
Potassium chloride 10 mEq 1 tab every morning

Hematological

Potassium chloride 10 mEq 1 tab every morning

Pulmonary

Be aware that some of the patient's medications may affect his respiratory effort.

Gastrointestinal

Atropine 0.3 mg every 4–6 hours as needed
Cholestyramine (Questran) 4 mg every morning
Potassium chloride 10 mEq 1 tab every morning
Chlordiazepoxide 5 mg every 8 hours
Allergies: Phenobarbital (PB); see explanation in the Neurological section.

Nutrition

The patient's major diagnosis was Crohn's disease, and most of his medications were centered on improving his nutritional status. This is a good example of medications being used in an off-label manner.

Genitourinary/renal

Sildenafil (Viagra) 25 mg 1 hour before sexual activity

Musculoskeletal

Ibuprofen 800 mg as needed for pain

Endocrine

None specific

Integumentary

None specific

Immune

The patient's major diagnosis was Crohn's disease, and most of his medications were centered on improving his nutritional status. Immunity may play a big part in the disease process.

Pain/comfort

Desvenlafaxine 50 mg
Ibuprofen, the drug specified for "pain"

Chlordiazepoxide 5 mg every 8 hours

Be aware that most medications were prescribed to alleviate the pain and discomfort of a disease process.

Nursing Process

☑ Self-Query: Possible Answers

The patient was diagnosed with a urinary tract infection and received Cipro. There was nothing visibly wrong with the ileostomy. More teaching was done, and he stated, "It will just take a while to adjust to this pouch; it really cramps my love life."

Case Study Inquiry

11

Vocabulary

Self-Query

Before attempting to work the case study, define each of the vocabulary words. Although the words may have several subheadings, it will give you a place to begin your inquiry.

Cirrhosis

_____

Diabetic ketoacidosis

_____

Hypoglycemia

_____

Hyperglycemic hyperosmolar nonketotic syndrome

_____

Pancreas

_____

Pancreatitis

_____

Type I diabetes mellitus

_____

Type II diabetes mellitus

_____

Your 68-year-old male patient has been admitted to home health following a 5-day stay in the hospital. Although he denied any past medical history (other than treatment for colon cancer), he was admitted from the emergency room with a blood sugar level of 600 and dehydration. After contacting his primary care provider, you discover that he has had numerous other health issues. He has been sent home on numerous medications, and he and his wife need assistance in setting a plan to monitor his medications.

Medications
Prehospital Medications

Calcium carbonate (Os-Cal) 500 D twice a day

Capecitabine (Xeloda) 500 mg twice a day

Furosemide (Lasix) 40 mg twice a day

Ibuprofen 200 mg before bedtime

Potassium 40 mEq twice a day

Posthospital Medications

Decrease potassium to 20 mEq once a day

Insulin glargine (Lantus) 55 units subcutaneously every night

Lisinopril 20 mg daily

Metformin 1000 mg every morning

⸮ Self-Query

Using a drug book or pharmacology text that contains the mechanism of action, unlabeled uses, and pharmacokinetics for medications, answer the following questions. Make answers specific to this scenario.

What do I know about these medications? Do I know the recommended dose of, the recommended route for, and the best time of day to give these medications? Do I know what lab results I need regarding each medication? Do I know the approved use of each medication? Do I know the most common diseases treated by the listed medications? Are any off-label uses approved for each drug?

Calcium carbonate

_____

_____

Capecitabine

_____

_____

Furosemide

_____

_____

Ibuprofen

_____

_____

Insulin glargine

_____

_____

Lisinopril

_____

_____

Metformin

_____

_____

Potassium

_____

_____

Do I know the individual's past medical history by looking at the medication list?

_____

_____

Allergies

Meperidine (Demerol)

Monosodium glutamate

Morphine

Self-Query

Do I know why each medication is used? Do I know the signs and symptoms of an adverse reaction to each medication? Do I know the classification of each medication?

Meperidine

_____

_____

Morphine

_____

_____

What is the metabolite of meperidine? What are the major side effects of the metabolite?

_____

Do I know where monosodium glutamate (MSG) is found? Why is it used?

_____

_____

Body Systems

Self-Query

Be prepared to defend your answers.

Can I place each medication under the body system that it commonly affects?

Neurological

_____

Cardiovascular

_____

Hematological

_____

Pulmonary

_____

Gastrointestinal

_____

Nutrition

_____

Genitourinary/renal

_____

Musculoskeletal

_____

Endocrine

Integumentary

Immune

Pain/comfort

Mechanism of Action

✌ Self-Query

Does the individual's medical history have an effect on the pharmacokinetics of each drug?

What contraindications do I need to address regarding the medications and medical history?

Nursing Process

✌ Self-Query

What nursing assessment will I perform regarding each medication? What planning and implementation do I need for each medication? How do I evaluate each medication's effectiveness?

Calcium carbonate

Capecitabine

Furosemide

Ibuprofen

Insulin glargine

Lisinopril

_____

_____

Metformin

_____

_____

Potassium

_____

_____

Do I need to be concerned about geriatric considerations with this individual?

_____

Follow-up

After 1 week at home, the patient's wife calls and states that her husband is "acting funny." You arrive at the home and find the following.

Assessment before calling ambulance:

The patient is confused. His skin is warm to the touch, heart rate 120, respirations 24, decreased breath sounds, coffee-ground emesis, and decreased bowel sounds. He is unable to lie flat without crying in pain. He is sent to the hospital and admitted to ICU.

Physical Assessment Findings

Neurological Assessment

Acute confusion and slurred speech; decreased consciousness; pupils equal, round, and reactive to light. Am I aware of how low or high the blood glucose must be before neurological symptoms appear?

Cardiovascular and Hematological Assessment

K+ 2.9, S_1S_2 monitor reveals sinus of 120.

Blood pressure 90/50, trace edema to extremities, pale, capillary refill at 3 seconds.

Pulmonary Assessment

Decreased breath sounds heard throughout; Kussmaul's rate 24 per minute on 4/L oxygen chest; X-ray reveals atelectasis.

Gastrointestinal Assessment

Decreased bowel sounds, poor dentations, guarding of abdomen > when the NGT was inserted, coffee-ground stomach contents were returned.

Weight: 135 pounds, height: 6'3".

Lab: amylase elevated, blood glucose 750, serum protein and calcium are low.

Genitourinary Assessment

Foley inserted, urine output at 150 mL/hour.

Musculoskeletal Assessment

Moving all extremities without problems.

Endocrine Assessment

HBA1C-10, pancreatic enzymes elevated.

Integumentary Assessment

Present IV to right antecubital, 0.9% NS at 150 mL/hr.

Immune Assessment

No palpable lymph nodes, no inflammation noted in joints.
Lab: WBC elevated.

Pain/Comfort Assessment

Grimace to abdominal assessment.

Physician ICU Orders

Calcium carbonate (Titralac) 1 g with water every 6 hours (6-12-6-12); may substitute with pharmacy formulary (per NGT)

Sucralfate (Carafate) 1 g every 6 hours (3-9-3-9) per NGT

Ondansetron (Zofran) 4 mg IV push every 6 hours as needed

Gentamicin 5mg/kg/day; divide over 4 doses

Hydromorphone (Dilaudid) 1–2 mg IV every 4 hours as needed for pain

Insulin infusion protocol (keep blood glucose 80–110)

Add 40 mEq KCL to each liter of NS

Consult nutrition and pharmacy for total parenteral nutrition (TPN) orders

❓ Self-Query

What do I know about these medications? For each medication, what is the recommended dose, recommended route, and best time of day to give it? Do I know what lab results I need in regard to each medication? Do I know why each of these medications was ordered for this patient?

Calcium carbonate

_____

_____

Sucralfate

_____

_____

Ondansetron

_____

_____

Gentamicin

_____

_____

Hydromorphone

_____

_____

Nursing Process

Self-Query

What nursing assessment will I perform regarding each medication? What planning and implementation do I need to do for each medication? How do I evaluate each medication's effectiveness?

Calcium carbonate

_____

_____

Sucralfate

_____

_____

Ondansetron

_____

_____

Gentamicin

_____

_____

Hydromorphone

_____

_____

Do I need to be concerned with geriatric considerations for this individual?

_____

What other medications might be needed in this situation? (Think acid–base balance and electrolytes.)

_____

_____

Synopsis

11

Because you can find answers to the self-queries in numerous texts, you will not find the answers to all of them here. However, you will find discussion of the individual case. The scenario relates to denial of endocrine/diabetes issues; therefore, purposefully look into the medication use and vocabulary as they relate to these issues.

Vocabulary

When reviewing the vocabulary words, you might want to ask several questions: who, what, where, when, why, and how. This should give you a much broader understanding of each word.

Do yourself a favor and do not just give the shortest and simplest answer. Use the following example of diabetic ketoacidosis (DKA): Instead of answering, "DKA is a complication in patients with diabetes mellitus," ask:

Who is most at risk for **diabetec ketoacidosis (DKA)**? How might DKA be induced by medications? Why is there dehydration in DKA? What is the treatment for DKA?

☑ Self-Query: Possible Answers

When defining the remainder of the vocabulary words, ask the following questions:

What is the pathophysiology of **cirrhosis**? Who is at risk for cirrhosis? How is cirrhosis medication induced? How is it lifestyle induced? What body system is altered?

What is **hypoglycemia**? How is hypoglycemia medication induced?

What is **hyperglycemic hyperosmolar nonketotic syndrome (HHNS)**? Who is at risk for HHNS? How is HHNS medication induced? What symptoms are seen in HHNS?

What is the **pancreas**? Explain how the pancreas is considered both an endocrine and exocrine gland.

What is the pathophysiology of **pancreatitis**? Who is at risk for pancreatitis? How is it medication related? How is it related to lifestyle?

What is the pathophysiology of diabetes? Who is at risk for **type I diabetes mellitus (DM)**? What are risk factors for the development of **type II DM**? How can type II DM be medication induced? What body system is affected?

Pre-ICU Medications

☑ Self-Query: Possible Answers

Neurological

> None of the patient's medications was classified as neurological. However, be aware that all the medications may have an effect on the patient's neurological status. The two medications for his diabetes are important from a neurological viewpoint. Under most circumstances, glucose is the sole source of energy for the brain.

Metformin 1000 mg every morning

Insulin glargine (Lantus) 55 units subcutaneously every night

Cardiovascular

Furosemide (Lasix) 40 mg twice a day
Potassium 40 mEq twice a day
Calcium carbonate (Os-Cal) 500+D twice a day
Lisinopril 20 mg daily

Hematological

Potassium 40 mEq twice a day

Calcium carbonate 500+D twice a day

Capecitabine (Xeloda) 500 mg twice a day. Capecitabine is taken daily for 2 weeks, followed by 1 week off the medication. The effect of capecitabine on this system may include anemia, neutropenia, and thrombocytopenia.

Pulmonary

None specific

Gastrointestinal

Calcium carbonate 500+D twice a day

Capecitabine 500 mg twice a day. Capecitabine is taken daily for 2 weeks, followed by 1 week off the medication. The administration is best if taken after a meal.

Nutrition

Potassium 40 mEq twice a day

Calcium carbonate 500+D twice a day

Capecitabine 500 mg 2 times a day. Capecitabine is taken daily for 2 weeks, followed by 1 week off the medication. The administration is best if taken after a meal.

Metformin 1000 mg every morning

Insulin glargine 55 units subcutaneously every night

Genitourinary/renal

Furosemide 40 mg twice a day
Ibuprofen 200 mg before bedtime (known to alter prostaglandins in the kidneys)
Calcium carbonate 500+D twice a day
Lisinopril 20 mg daily

Musculoskeletal

Ibuprofen 200 mg before bedtime
Calcium carbonate 500+D twice a day

Endocrine

Metformin 1000 mg every morning
Insulin glargine 55 units subcutaneously every night

Integumentary

Capecitabine 500 mg twice a day. Capecitabine is taken daily for 2 weeks, followed by 1 week off the medication. The administration is best if taken after a meal.

Capecitabine may cause hand and foot syndrome, also known as palmar-plantar erythema. This is a painful development of redness, tenderness, and possible peeling of the palms and soles. The first stage may appear as a sunburn. The areas affected can become dry and peel, with numbness or tingling developing. Capecitabine is placed under integumentary due to the effect it has on the skin such as dermatitis, alopecia, pruritus, hyperpigmentation, and other inflammatory responses of the skin.

Immune

Capecitabine 500 mg twice a day

Pain/comfort

You assess that there are no prescribed pain medications. Be aware that medications are prescribed to alleviate the pain and discomfort of the disease process.

Allergies: Meperidine (Demerol) and morphine are both pain medications. The metabolite is normeperidine, and it is metabolized primarily by the liver and excreted through the kidneys. Normeperidine is a cerebral irritant. MSG (monosodium glutamate) is made by a fermenting process using starch, sugar beets, sugar cane, or molasses. The patient stated that he experienced a headache, facial flushing and sweating, and difficulty breathing while eating at his favorite restaurant. This developed after his cancer therapy.

Physician ICU Orders

☑ Self-Query: Possible Answers

After consulting with the pharmacist, calcium carbonate (Titralac) was stopped and sucralfate (Carafate) was used.

Ondansetron (Zofran) is a **serotonin receptor antagonist** used mainly as an **antiemetic** to treat **nausea** and **vomiting** following **chemotherapy**. It is very effective in this case even though the nausea and vomiting were due in part to pancreatitis. Ondansetron reduces the activity on the **vagus nerve**, which activates the vomiting center in the **medulla oblongata**; it also blocks serotonin receptors in the **chemoreceptor trigger zone**.

Gentamicin 5mg/kg/day divided over 4 doses (used to prevent possible sepsis in pancreatitis).

Hydromorphone (Dilaudid) 1–2 mg IV every 4 hours as needed for pain; remember that the patient is allergic to meperidine and morphine.

Assessing and reviewing the A1C, the patient's HGA1C of 10 revealed that he had several months of pancreatic issues and elevated glucose levels.

Patient is dehydrated and has a potassium level of 2.9.

Consult nutrition and pharmacy for TPN orders.

Take into account that this patient is nauseated and has coffee-ground-appearing emesis. In addition, he is:

A cancer patient
A newly diagnosed diabetic
A person who denied any past medical history
A person who weighs 135 pounds and is 6'3"

The decision of whether to use the parenteral (IV) or enteral (GI) route for nutritional support was discussed with the physician. TPN allows maintenance of pancreatic rest. The role of enteral feedings is less clear. However, it has been shown that the further down the GI tract the feeding is infused, the less pancreatic stimulation occurs. Therefore, it seems wise to support the patient with TPN during severe acute pancreatitis. It is decided that enteral feedings should be initiated when the acute inflammatory phase ends.

Case Study Inquiry

12

Vocabulary

? Self-Query

Before attempting to work the case study, define each of the vocabulary words. Although the words may have several subheadings, it will give you a place to begin your inquiry.

Activities of daily living

_____

Adverse drug reactions

_____

Age-related pharmacokinetics

_____

B-type natriuretic peptide

_____

Drug–drug interactions

_____

Food–drug interactions

_____

Heart sounds (S_3 and S_4)

_____

Polypharmacy

_____

Purpura

_____

Serum medication levels

_____

Trough medication levels

_____

The 88-year-old female patient is in today for her yearly check-up. You are working in an office of a geriatric specialist. The patient's 70-year-old daughter is with her. You are reviewing the patient's medications. The patient states that she is not sleeping well and has lost weight because her appetite "just is not what it used to be."

Past Medical History

Atrial fibrillation, coronary artery disease, hyperlipidemia, hypertension, gout, gastroesophageal reflux disease, hyperthyroidism when she stwas 40 that went untreated for "a long time."

Home Medications

Acetaminophen (Tylenol) ES 2 tabs as needed for pain

Aspirin (ASA) 300 mg every morning orally

Furosemide (Lasix) 40 mg twice a day orally

Losartan (Cozaar) 50 mg daily

Metolazone (Zaroxolyn) 2.5 mg daily orally

Oxygen 2 L nasal cannula (wearing now)

Potassium 10 mEq twice a day orally

Warfarin (Coumadin) 1 mg daily

Self-Query

Using a drug book or pharmacology text that contains the mechanism of action, unlabeled uses, and pharmacokinetics for medications, answer the following questions. Make answers specific to this scenario.

What do I know about these medications? Do I know the recommended dose of, the recommended route for, and the best time of day to give these medications? Do I know what lab results I need regarding each medication? Do I know the approved use of each medication? Do I know the most common diseases treated by the listed medications? Are any off-label uses approved for each drug?

Acetaminophen

_____

_____

Aspirin

_____

_____

Furosemide

_____

_____

Losartan

_____

_____

Metolazone

_____

_____

Oxygen

_____

_____

Potassium

_____

_____

Warfarin

_____

_____

Are all the listed home medications necessary?

_____

Are there medications for each disease listed in the medical history?

_____

Body Systems

? Self-Query

Be prepared to defend your answers.

Can I place each medication under the body system that it commonly affects?

Neurological

_____

Cardiovascular

_____

Hematological

_____

Pulmonary

_____

Gastrointestinal

_____

Nutrition

_____

Genitourinary/renal

_____

Musculoskeletal

_____

Endocrine

_____

Integumentary

_____

Immune

_____

Pain/comfort

_____

Mechanism of Action

❓ Self-Query

Does the individual's medical history have an effect on the pharmacokinetics of the drug?

_____

_____

What contraindications do I need to address regarding the medications and medical history?

_____

_____

Nursing Process

❓ Self-Query

What nursing assessment will I perform regarding each medication? What planning and implementation do I need for each medication? How do I evaluate each medication's effectiveness?

Acetaminophen

_____

_____

Aspirin

_____

_____

Furosemide

_____

_____

Losartan

_____

_____

Metolazone

_____

_____

Oxygen

_____

_____

Potassium

_____

_____

Warfarin

_____

_____

Do I need to be concerned with any geriatric considerations for this individual?

_____

Physical Assessment Findings

Neurological Assessment

Alert, pleasant, talkative about family. Speech clear, appropriate responses appropriate for age.

Cardiac Assessment

Heart sounds $S_1S_2S_3$ irregular, cardiac monitor reveals atrial fibrillation with left-bundle branch block, distant heart sounds, radial pulses 2+ bilaterally, pedal pulses 1+ with noted 2+ edema to feet and lower legs. Blood pressure 102/50, heart rate 112, skin warm and dry, capillary refill < 3 seconds, moderate dyspnea at rest. Wearing oxygen at 2 L by nose prong.

Pulmonary Assessment

Respiratory rate 24, lungs with faint crackles

Gastrointestinal Assessment

Soft, nondistended abdomen, bowel sounds present in all quadrants. No reports of diarrhea or constipation; last bowel movement this morning.

Genitourinary Assessment

Slight stress incontinence (wears adult briefs). Urine specimen collected and revealed UTI.

Musculoskeletal Assessment

All extremities present with noted stiffening of connective tissue. Denies pain or soreness in joints.

Endocrine Assessment

No exophthalmia, no slow-healing wounds, no goiter; noted history of diabetes.

Integumentary Assessment

Skin warm to touch; patches of dry skin; no wounds, sores, or bruising noted.

Immune Assessment

No palpable lymph nodes.

Pain/Comfort Assessment

Denies pain at this time; states that she "took a pain pill this morning."

Physician Orders

Chest X-ray

CBC

PT/INR

B$_{12}$ level

Check to see if she received pneumonia vaccine

Ciprofloxacin (Cipro) 500 mg orally once daily for 10 days

❓ Self-Query

Why the vaccine? How often can it be administered? Does it matter what time of year it is given? How is it different from the influenza vaccine?

_____

_____

What classification is ciprofloxacin? What assessment finding would lead to the prescribing of ciprofloxacin?

_____

_____

Which medication is related to the PT/INR? What do you expect to find? What are the normal values of this test?

_____

_____

Why the B$_{12}$ level? If patient has a B$_{12}$ deficiency, how will it be treated? What will actually determine the medication and route for the deficiency?

_____

_____

You heard the physician discuss megestrol (Megace) with the patient and decide not to prescribe it. What in the medical history was a contraindication?

_____

_____

Synopsis

12

Because you can find answers to the self-queries in numerous texts, you will not find the answers to all of them here. However, you will find discussion of the individual case. The scenario relates to geriatrics and nutrition issues; therefore, purposefully look into the medication use and vocabulary as they relate to these issues.

Vocabulary

When reviewing the vocabulary words, you might want to ask several questions: who, what, where, when, why, and how. This should give you a much broader understanding of each word.

Do yourself a favor and do not just give the shortest and simplest answer. Use the following example of polypharmacy: Instead of answering, "Polypharmacy means that a person is using more than one drug," ask:

Who is at risk for **polypharmacy**? What causes polypharmacy? How can it be avoided?

☑ Self-Query: Possible Answers

When defining the remainder of the vocabulary words, ask the following questions:

How does one define **activities of daily living**? What are two examples of activities of daily living?

What is an **adverse drug reaction (ADR)**? How does the World Health Organization define an ADR? Who is at risk for ADRs? When is an ADR most likely to occur?

What are **age-related pharmacokinetics** (absorption, distribution, metabolism, excretion)? Who is most at risk for age-related pharmacokinetics?

What is a **B-type natriuretic peptide (BNP)**? Why is it measured? Where is it located? When is it significant? Who needs to have it measured?

What causes **drug–drug interactions**? Who is at risk for drug–drug interactions? What are two possible drug–drug consequences? How does aspirin (a drug) alter the levels of warfarin (a drug)?

What are **food–drug interactions**? What food would interfere with warfarin, monoamine oxidase inhibitors (MOAIs), and digoxin (Lanoxin)? Who is at risk for food–drug interactions? How does grapefruit juice affect certain medications?

What are **heart sounds**? What is an S_3 heart sound? When is an S_3 heard? What is an S_4 heart sound? When is an S_4 heard?

What is the pathophysiology of **purpura**? Who is at risk for purpura? Where is purpura located? How is it described?

What is a **serum medication level**? Why is it drawn? When is it drawn?

What is a **trough medication level**? Why is it drawn? When is it drawn?

Body Systems

☑ Self-Queries: Possible Answers

Neurological

Oxygen 2 L nasal cannula (wearing now)—the brain cannot survive without oxygen.

Cardiovascular

Oxygen 2 L nasal cannula (wearing now)
Aspirin (ASA) 300 mg every morning orally
Warfarin (Coumadin) 1 mg daily
Losartan (Cozaar) 50 mg daily
Potassium 10 mEq twice a day orally
Furosemide (Lasix) 40 mg twice a day orally
Metolazone (Zaroxolyn) 2.5 mg daily orally

Hematological

Oxygen 2 L nasal cannula (wearing now)
Aspirin 300 mg every morning orally
Warfarin 1 mg daily
Potassium 10 mEq twice a day orally
Metolazone 2.5 mg daily orally

Pulmonary

Oxygen 2 L nasal cannula (wearing now)
Pneumovax 23 0.5 mL in the deltoid muscle: The patient had not received the pneumococcal vaccine, so it was administered. Pneumococcal vaccination is a method of preventing a specific type of lung infection caused by the pneumococcal bacterium. Adults younger than 50 years of age without contraindications may be given 0.2 mL of an intranasal dose; 0.1 mL is sprayed into each nostril while the patient is in an upright position. Most people need to get it only once. It doesn't matter what time of year it is given. Influenza is seasonal and the vaccine is given yearly to certain populations. The pneumococcal vaccine is administered in the same fashion as the flu vaccine.
Ciprofloxacin (Cipro) 500 mg orally once daily for 10 days: It was prescribed for a UTI. However, there was a possibility of pneumonia. A chest x-ray revealed pneumonia, and because the patient had been prescribed ciprofloxacin for her UTI, nothing else was added. She was scheduled for a follow-up visit when the medication was completed. Be aware that any medication may affect this system, particularly in the geriatric individual.

Gastrointestinal

Although there are no specific medications related to this system, be aware that any medication may affect it, particularly in the geriatric individual.

Nutrition

Remember that the physician thought about prescribing megestrol (Megace) and then decided against it. Megestrol is progesterone, a hormone. Although Megestrol does increase the appetite and weight gain is thus secondary, the physician reviewed the chart and cardiac history. The other side effects—nausea, vomiting, edema, dyspnea, heart failure, hypertension, and mood changes—were more than the physician was willing to risk to have the patient gain a few pounds.

Remember these questions:

If patient has a B_{12} deficiency, how will it be treated? It depends on the cause of the deficiency.

The patient was diagnosed with pernicious anemia. Review the pathophysiology behind this. With any pathophysiology text, explore the connection among a decrease in the normal number of RBCs, a decreased amount of hemoglobin in the blood, and the intrinsic factor.

What will actually determine the medication and route for the deficiency? It depends on the cause of the deficiency. This patient was prescribed B_{12} injections, and home health was scheduled for the administration of this medication.

Genitourinary/renal

Furosemide 40 mg twice a day orally
Ciprofloxacin 500 mg orally once daily for 10 days
The patient's urine specimen revealed a UTI.

Musculoskeletal

Although there are no specific medications related to this system, be aware that any medication may affect it, particularly in the geriatric individual.

Endocrine

Did you assess that although the patient stated that she had thyroid problems, she was not taking any medication related to this?

Integumentary

Although there are no specific medications related to this system, be aware that any medication may affect it, particularly in the geriatric individual.

Immune

Although there are no specific medications related to this system, be aware that any medication may affect it, particularly in the geriatric individual.

Pain/comfort

Oxygen 2 L nasal cannula (wearing now)
Acetaminophen (Tylenol) ES 2 tabs as needed for pain
Be aware that although the following are not pain medications specifically, they are prescribed to decrease the discomfort of the disease process:
Aspirin 300 mg every morning orally
Warfarin 1 mg daily
Losartan 50 mg daily
Potassium 10 mEq twice a day orally
Furosemide 40 mg twice a day orally
Metolazone 2.5 mg daily orally

Case Study Inquiry

13

Vocabulary

Self-Query

Before attempting to work the case study, define each of the vocabulary words. Although the words may have several subheadings, it will give you a place to begin your inquiry.

Anticholinergic

_____

Cataract

_____

Clostridium difficile (C. difficile)

_____

Dehydration

_____

Erythrocytosis

_____

First-degree AV block

_____

Glomerular filtration rate

_____

Hyponatremia

_____

International normalized ratio (INR)

_____

Intrarenal insufficiency

_____

Jugular vein distention

_____

Mydriasis

_____

Osteoarthritis

_____

Pacemaker

_____

Pernicious anemia

_____

Postrenal failure

_____

Prerenal insufficiency

_____

Uremia

_____

An 83-year-old male called 911, stating that he could not stop vomiting and had diarrhea. Upon arrival to the emergency room, he reported abdominal cramping and experienced two diarrhea stools. He was sent immediately to your floor, where you have admitted him.

Past Medical History

Pacemaker for heart block, coronary stents, prerenal azotemia, pernicious anemia. You review the following laboratory results from the emergency room:

Negative for *C. difficile*; liver enzymes are within limits for his age.

Potassium 2.9; sodium 128, BUN 50, creatinine 2.0.

Home Medications

Aspirin (ASA) 325 mg every morning orally

Furosemide (Lasix) 40 mg twice a day orally

Ibuprofen (Motrin) 200 mg 2 tabs as needed for pain

Omega-3 two capsules every morning orally

Potassium 10 mEq twice a day orally

Vitamin B12

Self-Query

Using a drug book or pharmacology text that contains the mechanism of action, unlabeled uses, and pharmacokinetics for medications, answer the following questions. Make answers specific to this scenario.

What do I know about these medications? Do I know the recommended dose of, the recommended route for, and the best time of day to give these medications? Do I know what lab results I need regarding each medication? Do I know the approved use of each medication? Do I know the most common diseases treated by the listed medications? Are any off-label uses approved for each drug?

Aspirin

_____

_____

Furosemide

_____

_____

Ibuprofen

_____

_____

Omega-3

_____

_____

Potassium

_____

_____

Vitamin B12

_____

_____

There is no route or amount for this medication. Does this matter? What should the route be for this patient?

_____

Could any of the home medications have caused the extreme diarrhea and vomiting?

_____

Physician Orders

Nothing by mouth

IV normal saline at 125 mL/hr with 40 mEq potassium chloride (infusing from ER)

IV ondansetron (Zofran) 4 mL every 4 hours as needed (received 1 dose in ER)

Diphenoxylate hydrochloride and atropine sulfate (Lomotil) 5 mg orally as needed every 6 hours (received 1 dose in ER)

Oxygen 2 L nasal cannula, flat and upright

Place on telemetry

Obtain X-ray of abdomen (flat and upright)

May have clear liquid diet after X-ray cleared by radiologist

Self-Query

Do I know why each medication was ordered? Do I know the mechanism of action for each medication? Are there any factors in the individual's medical history that may affect the pharmacokinetics of each drug?

Normal saline with potassium chloride

_____

_____

Ondansetron

_____

_____

Diphenoxylate hydrochloride and atropine sulfate

_____

_____

Oxygen

_____

_____

What contraindications do I need to address regarding the medications and this individual's health history?

_____

_____

Nursing Process

Self-Query

What nursing assessment will I perform regarding each medication? What planning and implementation do I need to do for each medication? How do I evaluate each medication's effectiveness?

Normal saline with potassium chloride

_____

_____

Ondansetron

_____

_____

Diphenoxylate hydrochloride and atropine sulfate

_____

_____

Oxygen

_____

_____

Do I need to be concerned with geriatric considerations for this individual?

_____

_____

Follow-up

Your 83-year-old patient is recovering from his episode of vomiting and diarrhea and is feeling much better. As you walk down the hall with his son, you hear a loud crash in the man's room. Upon your arrival, the patient is lying on the floor in a supine position. You note quickly that the IV has been pulled out, urine and stool are on the floor, and blood is appearing from the back of the patient's head. The patient is lethargic. He is returned to the bed after assessment. A dressing is applied to the occipital area, and the IV is restarted.

Quick assessment: pupils 4+ sluggish reaction, bilaterally weak extremities, speech slurred.

The physician is contacted, and a CT of the head is ordered.

Report results revealed intracranial bleed.

The patient is transferred to neurological intensive care.

Vocabulary

Self-Query

Arachnoid membrane

_____

Cerebral perfusion pressure

_____

CT scan

_____

Decerebrate posturing

_____

Decorticate posturing

_____

Dura mater

_____

Glasgow coma scale

_____

MRI

_____

Pia mater

_____

Ventricular system

_____

Neurological Intensive Care Assessment

CT of head reveals:

Focal bleed to left cerebellum

Right subdural bleed with right posterior scalp edema

No midline shift, no skull fractures noted

Patient placed on a ventilator for respiratory support

Physician Orders

Over the next 2 days, the following medications are ordered before the family decides to make the patient a do not resuscitate (DNR):

Fentanyl citrate (Sublimaze) titrate dose as needed—supplied: fentanyl citrate 1000 mcg/20 mL in 100 mL of 5% dextrose

Propofol (Diprivan) titrate for sedation as needed—supplied: 1 gram in 100 mL (10 mg/mL)

IV ondansetron (Zofran) 4 mL every 4 hours as needed

Esomeprazole (Nexium) 40 mg IV every 24 hours

Lacri-Lube ophthalmic ointment every 8 hours

Chlorhexidine gluconate (Peridex) mouth care every shift

Mechanism of Action

℗ Self-Query

Do I know the mechanism of action for each medication? Are there any factors in the individual's medical history that may affect the pharmacokinetics of each drug?

Fentanyl citrate

_____

Propofol

_____

Ondansetron

_____

Esomeprazole

_____

Lacri-Lube

_____

Chlorhexidine gluconate

_____

What contraindications do I need to address regarding the medications and this individual's health history?

_____

_____

Nursing Process

Self-Query

What nursing assessment will I perform regarding each medication? What planning and implementation do I need to do for each medication? How do I evaluate each medication's effectiveness?

Fentanyl citrate

_____

_____

Propofol

_____

_____

Ondansetron

_____

_____

Esomeprazole

_____

_____

Lacri-Lube

_____

_____

Chlorhexidine gluconate

_____

_____

Are there any geriatric considerations for this individual?

_____

Do I know why these medications are prescribed to this man while he is on the ventilator?

_____

Synopsis

13

Because you can find answers to the self-queries in numerous texts, you will not find the answers to all of them here. However, you will find discussion of the individual case. The scenario relates to complications of a geriatric fall in the hospital and neurological issues; therefore, purposefully look into the medication use and vocabulary as they relate to these issues.

Vocabulary

When reviewing the vocabulary words, you might want to ask several questions: who, what, where, when, why, and how. This should give you a much broader understanding of each word.

Do yourself a favor and do not just give the shortest and simplest answer. Use the following example of a first-degree AV block: Instead of answering, "The AV block is a prolongation of the PR interval of the ECG beyond 0.20 seconds," ask:

Who develops a **first-degree AV block**? Why is it an important cardiac development? How is it caused by medications? How is it disease related?

☑ Self-Query: Possible Answers

When defining the remainder of the vocabulary words, ask the following questions:

How do **anticholinergics** alter kidney function?

What is a **cataract**?

What is *C. difficile*? Who is at risk for developing *C. difficile*? How is it treated?

How is **dehydration** diagnosed? Who is at risk for dehydration? Why is the person in the scenario at risk for dehydration?

What is the pathophysiology of **erythrocytosis**? Who is at risk for erythrocytosis?

What is the **glomerular filtration rate (GFR)**? Why is the GFR measured? How is GFR measured differently in the African American population? How does aspirin alter the GFR? What lab value reflects the GFR?

What is **hyponatremia**? Who is at risk for hyponatremia? How is it medication induced?

What is the **international normalized ratio (INR)**? How is it altered by warfarin (Coumadin)? Why is the value different for different diseases?

What are the causes of **intrarenal insufficiency**?

What causes **jugular vein distention (JVD)**? Who is at risk for JVD?

What is **mydriasis**? Who is at risk for mydriasis? How do certain medications alter the pupils? Which medications cause mydriasis?

What is the pathophysiology of **osteoarthritis**?

What is a **pacemaker**? Why are there different types? Who needs a pacemaker?

What is **pernicious anemia**? Who is at risk for pernicious anemia?

What are the causes of **postrenal failure**?

What are the causes of **prerenal insufficiency**?

How is **uremia** treated? Who is at risk for uremia?

Body Systems

☑ Self-Query: Possible Answers

Neurological

The 83-year-old man had no prescriptions for any neurological condition. Be aware of the mechanism of action of IV ondansetron (Zofran) 4 mL every 4 hours PRN (he received 1 dose in the ER).

Cardiovascular

Aspirin (ASA) 325 mg every morning orally
Potassium 10 mEq twice a day orally
Furosemide (Lasix) 40 mg twice a day orally
Omega-3 two capsules every morning orally
Oxygen 2 L nasal cannula
B12 (need to find dose, route, and time; this is determined by the type of anemia)

Pulmonary

Oxygen 2 L nasal cannula

Gastrointestinal

Be aware of the mechanism of action of IV ondansetron 4 mL every 4 hours as needed (received 1 dose in ER).
Vitamin B12 (you would need to retrieve the route, dose, times)
IV normal saline at 125 mL/hr with 40 mEq potassium chloride
IV ondansetron 4 mL every 4 hours as needed (acts on the neurological system)
Diphenoxylate hydrochloride and atropine sulfate (Lomotil) 5 mg orally as needed every 6 hours (Can you explain why these two medications are combined?)

Genitourinary

Patient had no medications prescribed specifically for this system.
IV normal saline at 125 mL/hr with 40 mEq potassium chloride
Think how this would decrease the possibility of renal failure caused by dehydration.

Musculoskeletal

Ibuprofen (Motrin) 200 mg 2 tabs as needed for pain
IV normal saline at 125 mL/hr with 40 mEq potassium chloride

Endocrine

The patient had medications prescribed specifically for this system.

Integumentary

The patient had medications prescribed specifically for this system.
IV normal saline at 125 mL/hr with 40 mEq potassium chloride

Immune

The patient had medications prescribed specifically for this system.

Pain/comfort

Ibuprofen 200 mg 2 tabs as needed for pain. Ibuprofen may interfere with the cardiac effects of aspirin.

IV normal saline at 125 mL/hr with 40 mEq potassium chloride

IV ondansetron 4 mL every 4 hours as needed (acts on the neurological system)

Follow-up

The patient suffers a fall and complications and is transferred to the neurological ICU.

Vocabulary

☑ Self-Query: Possible Answers

What is the **arachnoid membrane**? Where is the arachnoid membrane located?

What is the **cerebral perfusion pressure**? What is the normal pressure? How is it calculated?

Why use a **CT scan**? How is a CT scan different from an MRI?

What is the pathophysiology of **decerebate posturing**? Who is at risk for decerebrate posturing? How is it treated?

What is the pathophysiology of **decorticate posturing**? Who is at risk for decorticate posturing? How is it treated?

What is the dura mater? Where is the **dura mater** located?

What is the **Glasgow coma scale**? How is it evaluated?

Why use an **MRI**? How is an MRI different from a CT scan?

What is the **pia mater**? Where is the pia mater located?

What is the **ventricular system** of the brain? How many ventricles does the brain have?

Body Systems

☑ Self-Query: Possible Answers

Neurological

Fentanyl citrate (Sublimaze) titrate dose as needed
Propofol titrate (Diprivan) as needed
IV ondansetron 4 mL every 4 hours as needed

Gastrointestinal

Esomeprazole (Nexium) 40 mg IV every 24 hours

Pain/comfort

Lacri-Lube ophthalmic ointment every 8 hours
Chlorhexidine gluconate (Peridex) mouth care every shift

This is a grim reminder of the danger of falls. The patient remained on the ventilator for 3 days before being made a DNR. The ventilator was removed, and he died within the hour.

Case Study Inquiry

14

Vocabulary

? Self-Query

Before attempting to work the case study, define each of the vocabulary words. Although the words may have several subheadings, it will give you a place to begin your inquiry.

Abdominal wound dehiscence

_____

Colon

_____

Disseminated intravascular coagulation (DIC)

_____

Duodenum

_____

Jejunum

_____

Ileum

_____

Morbid obesity

_____

Peptic ulcer disease

_____

Pulmonary embolus

_____

Sepsis

_____

You are attempting to do an assessment on a 55-year-old female brought into the emergency room by ambulance. Her husband arrived home from work and found her confused, short of breath, and complaining of severe abdominal and chest pain.

Recent History

The patient underwent abdominal surgery 6 weeks ago. She has experienced nausea and vomiting over the past few days. She visited the emergency room 3 days ago and complained of fever (100.1°F), cough, and general malaise. No other labs were drawn. She was prescribed amoxicillin. She informed her husband this morning that she was feeling better. He found his wife "just like this," pointing to her lying on the stretcher.

Home Medications

Per the patient's husband:

Acetaminophen and propoxyphene (Darvocet-N 100) orally as needed for pain

Amoxicillin (Amoxil) 500 mg every 8 hours orally

Diazepam (Valium) 5 mg orally as needed for pain

Furosemide (Lasix) 40 mg daily orally

Metoprolol (Lopressor) 50 mg daily orally

Multivitamin with Fe+

Omeprazole (Prilosec) 20 mg daily orally

Tizanidine (Zanaflex) 2 mg orally daily

Tramadol (Ultram) 50 mg orally 3 times a day

Self-Query

Using a drug book or pharmacology text that contains the mechanism of action, unlabeled uses, and pharmacokinetics for medications, answer the following questions. Make answers specific to this scenario.

What do I know about these medications? Do I know the recommended dose of, the recommended route for, and the best time of day to give these medications? Do I know what lab results I need regarding each medication? Do I know the approved use of each medication? Do I know the most common diseases treated by the listed medications? Are any off-label uses approved for each drug?

Acetaminophen and propoxyphene

_____

_____

Amoxicillin

_____

_____

Diazepam

_____

_____

Furosemide

_____

_____

Metoprolol

_____

_____

Multivitamin with Fe+

_____

_____

Omeprazole

_____

_____

Tizanidine

_____

_____

Tramadol

_____

_____

What does the N-100 signify in the Darvocet?

_____

Do I know why the patient is on acetaminophen and propoxyphene, tramadol, and diazepam at the same time?

_____

_____

Allergies

Codeine

Lisinopril (Prinivil)

Sulfa

Self-Query

Do I know which sulfa medication was most likely prescribed in the patient's past? Do I know the classification of sulfa, and can I name a common sulfa drug? Do I know the signs and symptoms of an adverse reaction to sulfa?

_____

_____

Do I know why each medication was most likely prescribed in the past? Do I know the signs and symptoms of an adverse reaction to each medication? Do I know the classification of each medication?

Codeine

_____

_____

Lisinopril

_____

_____

What is codeine's most common side effect? In relation to codeine, are there other medications in this classification that are more likely to cause an allergy?

_____

_____

Body Systems I

Self-Query

Be prepared to defend your answers.

Can I place each medication under the body system that it commonly affects?

Neurological

_____

Cardiovascular

_____

Hematological

_____

Pulmonary

_____

Gastrointestinal

_____

Nutrition

_____

Genitourinary/renal

_____

Musculoskeletal

_____

Endocrine

_____

Integumentary

_____

Immune

_____

Pain/comfort

_____

Mechanism of Action

❓ Self-Query

Does the individual's medical history have an effect on the pharmacokinetics of each drug?

_____

_____

What contraindications do I need to address regarding the medications and medical history?

_____

_____

Nursing Process

❓ Self-Query

What nursing assessment will I perform regarding each medication? What planning and implementation do I need to do for each medication? How do I evaluate each medication's effectiveness?

Acetaminophen and propoxyphene

_____

_____

Amoxicillin

_____

_____

Diazepam

_____

_____

Furosemide

_____

_____

Metoprolol

_____

_____

Multivitamin with Fe+

_____

_____

Omeprazole

_____

_____

Tizanidine

_____

_____

Tramadol

_____

_____

Do I need to be concerned about geriatric considerations with this individual?

_____

Physical Assessment Findings

Neurological Assessment

Pupils equal, round, and sluggishly reactive to light. Responsive to verbal stimuli but not appropriate.

Cardiovascular and Hematological Assessment

S_1S_2 monitor reveals sinus tachycardia 112

Blood pressure 210/100, extremities pale, 3+ pitting edema

Capillary refill at 3 seconds

No JVD; no murmurs, gallops, or rubs

BNP 973; CK-MB 3.3; potassium 6.0; platelets 100,000

Pulmonary Assessment

Decreased lung sounds throughout, respiratory rate 24 per minute

Oxygen 2 L/min O_2 sat 94%

Symmetrical chest movements

Gastrointestinal Assessment

Large, separating abdominal wound

Weight presently 136 kg, hypoactive bowel sounds

Mouth with poor dentition, crusted food to roof of mouth

Labs: alkaline phosphate 276; albumin 1.1; SGOT 50; SGPT 40; blood glucose 400

Genitourinary Assessment

Foley inserted; 100 mL of dark, concentrated urine returned

Musculoskeletal Assessment

Husband reports history of arthritis

Able to move all extremities

Endocrine Assessment

No exophthalmia, no goiter

Integumentary Assessment

Open wound to mid-abdominal area, noted dark necrotic tissue around wound

Foul smelling drainage from wound

IV site to right antecubital 0.9% NS at 100 mL/hr

Immune Assessment

No palpable lymph nodes

Pain/Comfort Assessment

Moaning and groaning when entire abdominal area is palpated

Physician Orders

Before transfer to the critical care unit, the emergency room physician writes the following:

Assessment impression:

    Sepsis r/t large abdominal wound

    Acute renal failure

Hyperkalemia

Hypertension

Hyperglycemia

Anemia

Elevated liver enzyme

Malnutrition

Transfer to critical care with the following orders:

Nothing by mouth and discontinue home meds

Transfuse 2 units packed RBCs

Insulin drip protocol titrate to keep blood glucose between 80 and 110

Piperacillin and tazobactam (Zosyn) 3.375 g every 6 hours IV

Vancomycin 2000 mg every 8 hours IV

Albumin 5% IV every 24 hours

Labetalol (Normodyne) 200 mg slow IV push

Self-Query

Why were the packed RBCs ordered?

_____

What are the nursing interventions regarding the insulin drip?

_____

What are the classifications of the two antibiotics, and why were both prescribed?

_____

_____

What is the reason for the albumin, and what is its classification?

_____

_____

How will you know that each medication has worked?

_____

_____

What are the nursing interventions related to labetalol?

_____

Critical Care Physician Orders

During the second blood transfusion, the patient developed respiratory failure and was intubated. The patient is now on the ventilator with the following additional orders:

Fentanyl (Sublimaze) titrate for sedation as needed—supplied: fentanyl citrate 1000 mcg/20 mL in 100 mL of 5% dextrose

Propofol (Diprivan) titrate as needed—supplied: 1 gram in 100 mL (10 mg/mL)

Lorazepam (Ativan) 25 mg drip over 24 hours—supplied: 25 mg in 250 mL of NS

IV ondansetron (Zofran) 4 mL every 4 hours as needed

Acetaminophen (Tylenol) 650 mg rectal suppository every 4 hours as needed T. > 100.0°F

Esomeprazole (Nexium) 40 mg IV every 24 hours

Lacri-Lube ophthalmic ointment every 8 hours

Chlorhexidine gluconate (Peridex) mouth care every shift

Enoxaparin (Lovenox) 30 mg subcutaneously every 12 hours

Ceftriaxone (Rocephin) 2 grams IV every 12 hours

Body Systems II

? Self-Query

Be prepared to defend your answers.

Can I place each medication under the body system that it commonly affects?

Neurological

_____

Cardiovascular

_____

Hematological

_____

Pulmonary

_____

Gastrointestinal

_____

Nutrition

_____

Genitourinary/renal

_____

Musculoskeletal

_____

Endocrine

_____

Integumentary

_____

Immune

_____

Pain/comfort

_____

Nursing Process

? Self-Query

What nursing assessment will I do regarding each medication? What planning and implementation do I need to do for each medication? How do I evaluate each medication's effectiveness?

Insulin

_____

_____

Piperacillin and tazobactam

_____

_____

Vancomycin

_____

_____

Albumin

_____

_____

Labetalol

_____

_____

Fentanyl

_____

_____

Propofol

_____

_____

Lorazepam

_____

_____

Ondansetron

_____

_____

Acetaminophen

_____

_____

Esomeprazole

_____

_____

Lacri-Lube

_____

_____

Chlorhexidine gluconate

_____

_____

Enoxaparin

_____

_____

Ceftriaxone

What orders are related to the ventilator bundle?

What lab results are needed for the propofol?

What lab results are needed for the ceftriaxone?

How do these medications relieve pain and increase comfort?

Synopsis

14

Because you can find answers to the self-queries in numerous texts, you will not find the answers to all of them here. However, you will find discussion of the individual case. The scenario relates to abdominal infection; therefore, purposefully look into the medication use and vocabulary as they relate to abdominal infections.

Vocabulary

When reviewing the vocabulary words, you might want to ask several questions: who, what, where, when, why, and how. This should give you a much broader understanding of the word.

Do yourself a favor and do not just give the shortest and simplest answer. Use the following example of duodenum: Instead of answering, "The duodenum is part of the small intestine connecting the rest of the intestine to the stomach," ask:

Why is the **duodenum** important? What diseases most alter the duodenum? What medications are dissolved in this portion of the small intestine?

☑ Self-Query: Possible Answers

When defining the remainder of the vocabulary words, ask the following questions:

What causes an **abdominal wound dehiscence**?

Why is the **colon** important? What diseases most alter the function of the colon? What medications are dissolved in this portion of the intestine? How is bacteria beneficial and also harmful in the gastrointestinal tract?

What is the pathophysiology of **disseminated intravascular coagulation (DIC)**? Who is at risk for DIC? What medications are used in the treatment of DIC?

Why is the **jejunum** important? What diseases most alter the jejunum? What medications are dissolved in this portion of the small intestine?

Why is the **ileum** important? What diseases most alter the ileum? What medications are dissolved in this portion of the small intestine? Where are enteric-coated medications dissolved?

What causes **morbid obesity**? What medications are used to treat morbid obesity? What are the parameters for classing someone as morbidly obese?

What is the pathophysiology of **peptic ulcer disease**? Where are peptic ulcers located? What medications are used to treat this disease?

What causes a **pulmonary embolus**? What medications are used in the treatment of a pulmonary embolus? Who is at risk for a pulmonary embolus?

What is the pathophysiology of **sepsis**? Who is at risk for sepsis? What medications are used in sepsis?

Home Medications

☑ Self-Query: Possible Answers

Several medications need to be reviewed. The patient has several medications that are used for the same disorders. More questions need to be asked.

Body Systems I

☑ Self-Query: Possible Answers

Neurological

>   Acetaminophen and propoxyphene (Darvocet-N 100)—an analog of codeine (How does this relate to the patient's codeine allergy?)
>
>   Tizanidine (Zanaflex) 2 mg orally daily—usually associated with sedation
>
>   Diazepam (Valium) 5 mg orally as needed—usually associated with sedation

Cardiac

>   Furosemide (Lasix) 40 mg daily orally
>
>   Metoprolol (Lopressor) 50 mg daily orally

Hematology

>   Multivitamin with Fe+

Pulmonary

>   None specific
>
>   Amoxicillin (Amoxil) 500 mg every 8 hours orally
>
>   It is difficult to decide which system this affects because it was prescribed in the emergency room after the patient reported cough, general malaise, and low-grade fever during a previous visit.

Gastrointestinal

>   Omeprazole (Prilosec) 20 mg daily orally

Nutritional

>   The case does not say if the surgery was gastric bypass, or indeed what type of surgery was performed.
>
>   Multivitamin with Fe+

Genitourinary

>   None specific

Musculoskeletal

>   Tizanidine 2 mg orally daily—usually associated with sedation
>
>   Diazepam 5 mg orally as needed—usually associated with sedation

Endocrine

>   None specific

Integumentary

>   None specific

Immune

>   None specific

Pain/comfort

>   Acetaminophen and propoxyphene
>
>   Tramadol (Ultram) 50 mg orally 3 times a day—an analog of codeine (How does this relate to the patient's codeine allergy?)

Tizanidine 2 mg orally daily—usually associated with sedation
Diazepam 5 mg orally as needed—usually associated with sedation

Body Systems II

☑ Self-Query: Possible Answers

Neurological

Fentanyl (Sublimaze) titrate to patient's needs
Propofol (Diprivan) titrate to patient's needs
Lorazepam (Ativan) 25-mg drip over 24 hours
IV ondansetron (Zofran) 4 mL every 4 hours as needed

Cardiovascular

Fentanyl
Albumin 5% IV every 24 hours
Labetalol (Normodyne) 200 mg slow IV push (see blood pressure on assessment)—20 mg was infused over 2 minutes. After 10 minutes, there was no decrease; an additional 40 mg was given, and another 40 mg 10 minutes later. This was repeated until 200 mg was given. The pressure decreased to 130/88 from 210/100.
Transfuse 2 units packed RBCs (each infused over 4 hours with 40 mg IV furosemide before each infusion).

Hematological

Transfuse 2 units packed RBCs
Albumin 5% IV every 24 hours
Enoxaparin (Lovenox) 30 mg subcutaneously every 12 hours

Pulmonary

Oxygen 2 L (Remember to consider oxygen a medication.)

Gastrointestinal

Piperacillin and tazobactam (Zosyn) 3.375 gm every 6 hours IV
Vancomycin 2000 mg every 8 hours IV
Esomeprazole (Nexium) 40 mg IV every 24 hours
Ceftriaxone (Rocephin) 2 g IV every 12 hours

Nutrition

Insulin drip protocol titrate to keep blood glucose between 80 and 110

Genitourinary/renal

IV ondansetron 4 mL every 4 hours as needed
Her hyperkalemia was related to prerenal hypovolemia. You do not have a creatinine level; however, assessment of her other lab results would make you think it was also elevated.

Musculoskeletal

Fentanyl titrate to patient's needs
Propofol titrate to patient's needs
Lorazepam 25 mg drip over 24 hours

Endocrine

Insulin drip protocol titrate to keep blood glucose between 80 and 110

Integumentary (note the integumentary assessment)

Piperacillin and tazobactam 3.375 gm every 6 hours IV
Vancomycin 2000 mg every 8 hours IV
Ceftriaxone 2 g IV every 12 hours

Immune

No medications to boost immunity.

Pain/comfort

Note that medications do not have to be "pain" medications to relieve pain and increase comfort.
Transfuse 2 units packed RBCs
Insulin drip protocol titrate to keep blood glucose between 80 and 110
Piperacillin and tazobactam 3.375 gm every 6 hours IV
Vancomycin 2000 mg every 8 hours IV
Albumin 5% IV every 24 hours
Labetalol 200 mg 200 mg slow IV push
Fentanyl titrate to patient's needs—supplied: fentanyl citrate 1000 mcg/20 mL in 100 mL of 5% dextrose
Propofol titrate to patient's needs—supplied: 1 gram in 100 mL (10 mg/mL)
Lorazepam 25 mg drip over 24 hours—supplied: 25 mg in 250 mL of normal saline
IV ondansetron 4 mL every 4 hours as needed
Acetaminophen (Tylenol) 650 mg rectal suppository every 4 hours as needed T. > 100.0°F
Esomeprazole 40 mg IV every 24 hours
Lacri-Lube ophthalmic ointment every 8 hours
Chlorhexidine gluconate (Peridex) mouth care every shift
Enoxaparin 30 mg subcutaneously every 12 hours
Ceftriaxone 2 g IV every 12 hours

Nursing Process

☑ Self-Query: Possible Answers

The patient had undergone abdominal surgery on her gallbladder. There was a small laceration in the bowel, and it was not discovered until the patient was home and began to recover. The incision did not heal properly because of several factors: her weight of 136 kg, undiagnosed type II diabetes mellitus, and poor nutritional support.

You may want to discuss the implications of not only the medications but also the possible outcome of a person of this size on a ventilator who developed septic shock.

Ventilator bundle (you may want to look up evidence-based results regarding this)
Stress ulcer prophylaxis—esomeprazole 40 mg IV every 24 hours
DVT prophylaxis—enoxaparin 30 mg subcutaneously every 12 hours
Needed propofol lab: Liver enzymes should be monitored because it is supplied in a mixture of soybean oil, glycerol, and egg lecithin.
Needed ceftriaxone lab: This drug was chosen because it is only one of two cephalosporins that does not require dosage reduction in person with renal impairment.

The patient did not survive the sepsis.

Case Study Inquiry

15

Vocabulary

❓ Self-Query

Before attempting to work the case study, define each of the vocabulary words. Although the words may have several subheadings, it will give you a place to begin your inquiry.

Anemia

_____

Benign prostatic hypertrophy

_____

Beta receptor

_____

Dyspnea

_____

Insomnia

_____

Lumbago

_____

Nocturia

_____

Orthopnea

_____

Platelet aggregation

_____

Spinal stenosis

_____

The patient, an 80-year-old African American male, is in today because he says he has not had a bowel movement in a week, and he wants his healthcare provider to "do something." His daughter states that she has brought her father in because she noticed he had a fever of 100.6°F and a productive cough. You have completed your assessment and are reviewing the patient's medications. He has given you a brown paper bag with his medicines. He tells you, "I keep all my medications together."

Past Medical History

Depression, chronic kidney failure, lumbago, gastroesophageal reflux disease, benign prostate hypertrophy (BPH), insomnia, anemia, cerebrovascular accident, hypertension, hyperlipidemia.

Home Medications

Amlodipine besylate (Norvasc) 10 mg orally

Aspirin and dipyridamole (Aggrenox) 1 capsule daily

Atenolol (Tenormin) 50 mg orally daily

Bumetanide (Bumex) 2 mg 1 tab twice daily

Docusate (Colace) 100 mg orally at bedtime

Doxazosin (Cardura) 4 mg 1 tab twice a day

Eucerin apply to skin as needed

Furosemide (Lasix) 20 mg orally every morning

Isosorbide (Imdur) 60 mg orally daily

Sennosides (Senokot) 2 tabs every morning for constipation

Self-Query

Using a drug book or pharmacology text that contains the mechanism of action, unlabeled uses, and pharmacokinetics for medications, answer the following questions. Make answers specific to this scenario.

What do I know about these medications? For each medication, what is the recommended dose, recommended route, and best time of day to give it? Do I know what lab results I need in regard to each medication? Do I know the approved use of each medication? Do I know the most common diseases treated by the listed medications? Are any off-label uses approved for each drug?

Amlodipine besylate

_____

_____

Aspirin and dipyridamole

_____

_____

Atenolol

_____

_____

Bumetanide

_____

_____

Docusate

_____

_____

Doxazosin

_____

_____

Eucerin

_____

_____

Furosemide

_____

_____

Isosorbide

_____

_____

Sennosides

_____

_____

Are all the medications necessary?

_____

Are there medications for each disease listed in the medical history? (Explain your answer.)

_____

_____

If some of the medications are duplicates, how will you discuss this with the patient?

_____

If some of the medications are duplicates, how you will discuss this with the physician?

_____

Body Systems

? Self-Query

Be prepared to defend your answers.

Can I place each medication under the body system that it commonly affects?

Neurological

_____

Cardiovascular

_____

Hematological

_____

Pulmonary

_____

Gastrointestinal

_____

Nutrition

_____

Genitourinary/renal

_____

Musculoskeletal

_____

Endocrine

_____

Integumentary

_____

Immune

_____

Pain/comfort

_____

Mechanism of Action

? Self-Query

Does the individual's medical history have an effect on the pharmacokinetics of each drug?

_____

_____

What contraindications do I need to address regarding the medications and medical history?

_____

_____

Nursing Process

? Self-Query

What nursing assessment will I do regarding each medication? What planning and implementation do I need to conduct for each medication? How do I evaluate each medication's effectiveness?

Amlodipine besylate

_____

_____

Aspirin and dipyridamole

_____

_____

Atenolol

_____

_____

Bumetanide

_____

_____

Docusate

_____

_____

Doxazosin

_____

_____

Eucerin

_____

_____

Furosemide

_____

_____

Isosorbide

_____

_____

Sennosides

_____

_____

Do I need to be concerned about geriatric considerations with this individual?

_____

Physical Assessment Findings

Neurological Assessment

The patient states that he has a decreased energy level and is not always able to walk his small dog. His daughter has noticed that he has an unsteady gait when walking from the living room couch to the table to eat. Slight tremors when setting quietly are noted; his speech is clear. He is concerned about constipation and does not know why his daughter has brought him to the clinic.

Cardiac Assessment

Heart sounds S_1S_2; ECG reveals atrial fibrillation with left-bundle branch block; distant heart sounds; radial pulses 2+ bilaterally; pedal pulses 1+ with noted 2+ edema to feet and lower legs. Blood pressure 200/110, heart rate 118, skin warm and dry, capillary refill >3 seconds.

Pulmonary Assessment

Respiratory rate 24, lungs with bilateral crackles

Gastrointestinal Assessment

Firm distended abdomen, bowel sounds hyperactive in all quadrants. The patient reports constipation. He states that his last bowel movement "seems like a month ago"; he cannot remember last bowel movement ("but not today").

Genitourinary Assessment

The patient's daughter states that he has an overactive bladder and wears adult briefs.

Musculoskeletal Assessment

Noted stiffness in movement; reports pain in hands and feet.

Endocrine Assessment

No exophthalmia, no slow-healing wounds, and no goiter; noted history of diabetes.

Integumentary Assessment

Skin warm to touch; patches of dry, scaly skin; no wounds or sores; no bruising noted. Red rash on buttocks and backs of thighs.

Immune Assessment

No palpable lymph nodes.

Pain/Comfort Assessment

The patient states that the only problem is the need for a bowel movement.

Physician Orders

After the physician assessment, note following orders:

Admit to medical floor

Chest X-ray

KUB

MRI of head

PT/INR

CBC

Metabolic profile

CRP/BNP

IV NS 100 mL/hr

If potassium less than 3.5, begin KCL 40 mEq to each bag of NS

Medical Floor Physician Orders

Atenolol (Tenormin) 50 mg orally daily

Amlodipine besylate (Norvasc) 10 mg orally daily

Aspirin and dipyridamole (Aggrenox) 1 capsule daily orally

Bumetanide (Bumex) 2 mg 1 tab twice daily orally

Clonidine (Catapres) 0.1 mg 1 tab twice a day orally

Doxazosin (Cardura) 4 mg 1 tab twice a day orally

Eucerin apply to skin as needed

Imipenem and cilastatin (Primaxin) 250 mg IV every 8 hours

Isosorbide (Imdur) 60 mg orally daily

Polyethylene glycol (MiraLax) 1 tsp orally only after results of KUB

Self-Query

Are there any changes? If so, why?

_____

_____

Are there still medications that need to be reviewed with the physician?

_____

What classification is imipenem and cilastatin? Why is it given? How is it given?

_____

_____

Do I know why the physician ordered Cipro for this individual?

_____

Synopsis

15

Because you can find answers to the self-queries in numerous texts, you will not find the answers to all of them here. However, you will find discussion of the individual case. The scenario relates to a geriatric individual with reports of constipation, a cough, and a fever; therefore, purposefully look into the medication use and vocabulary as they relate to these factors.

Vocabulary

When reviewing the vocabulary words, you might want to ask several questions: who, what, where, when, why, and how. This should give you a much broader understanding of each word.

Do yourself a favor and do not just give the shortest and simplest answer. Use the following example of benign prostate hypertrophy (BPH): Instead of answering, "Benign prostate hypertrophy is an enlarged prostate that is not cancerous," ask:

Why is the prostate important? Who is at risk for **benign prostate hypertrophy (BPH)**? What medications cause BPH? What medications relieve BPH?

☑ Self-Query: Possible Answers

When defining the remainder of the vocabulary words, ask the following questions:

What is **anemia**? What are the causes of anemia? Who is at risk for anemia? What makes this individual at risk for anemia? What are the different treatments for anemia? What medications are used to treat anemia?

What are **beta receptors**? Where are beta receptors located? How are beta receptors affected by medications? Which body systems are most affected by these medications?

What is **dyspnea**? What are the causes of dyspnea? Who is at risk for dyspnea? What makes this individual at risk for dyspnea? What are the different treatments for dyspnea? What medications are used to treat dyspnea?

What is **insomnia**? Is it more prevalent in the geriatric population? Which medications can cause insomnia? Which medications relieve insomnia? Why is this individual at risk for insomnia?

What is **lumbago**? Where is it located? Who is at risk for lumbago? What are the treatments for lumbago?

What is **nocturia**? Who is at risk for nocturia? What medical condition makes this individual at risk?

What is **orthopnea**? What are the causes of orthopnea? Who is at risk for orthopnea? What makes this individual at risk for orthopnea? What are the different treatments for orthopnea? What medications are used to treat orthopnea? How do dyspnea and orthopnea differ?

What is **platelet aggregation**? What are the causes of platelet aggregation? Who is at risk for platelet aggregation? Is this a good thing or not? What medications are used to affect platelet aggregation?

What is **spinal stenosis**? What part of the spine is usually affected? Who is at risk for spinal stenosis? What are the treatments for spinal stenosis?

Home Medications

Depression—no medications

Chronic kidney failure

    Furosemide 20 mg orally every morning
    Bumetanide (Bumex) 2 mg 1 tab twice daily
    Eucerin apply to skin as needed

Lumbago—no medication

Gastroesophageal reflux disease—no medication

Benign prostate hypertrophy—no medication

Insomnia—no medication

Anemia—no medication

Cerebrovascular accident: R/T hypertension

    Isosorbide 60 mg orally daily
    Aspirin and dipyridamole (Aggrenox) 1 capsule daily

Hypertension

    Isosorbide 60 mg orally daily
    Atenolol 50 mg orally daily
    Amlodipine besylate (Norvasc) 10 mg orally
    Doxazosin (Cardura) 4 mg 1 tab twice a day

Hyperlipidemia—no medication

In summary, there are not medications for each disease, and the bumetanide and furosemide (Lasix) are drugs from the same category: one of them is not needed.

Body Systems

✓ Self-Query: Possible Answers

Neurological

None

Cardiovascular

    Furosemide 20 mg orally every morning (edema)
    Isosorbide (Imdur) 60 mg orally daily
    Atenolol (Tenormin) 50 mg orally daily
    Amlodipine besylate 10 mg orally
    Aspirin and dipyridamole 1 capsule daily
    Bumetanide 2 mg 1 tab twice daily
    Doxazosin 4 mg 1 tab twice a day

Hematological

    Aspirin and dipyridamole 1 capsule daily

Pulmonary

None

Gastrointestinal

Senokot 2 tabs every morning for constipation
Docusate (Colace) 100 mg orally at bedtime

Nutrition

None

Genitourinary/renal

Furosemide 20 mg orally every morning
Bumetanide 2 mg 1 tab twice daily

Musculoskeletal

None

Endocrine

None

Integumentary

Eucerin apply to skin as needed

Immune

None

Pain/comfort

No pain medications; however, keep in mind that his medications are to promote comfort and pain relief.

Medical Floor Physician Orders

☑ Self-Query: Possible Answers

Most medications were continued.

The furosemide was stopped and the bumetanide continued.

Clonidine (Catapres) 0.1 mg was added for blood pressure.

Polyethylene glycol (MiraLax) 1 tsp was ordered after KUB was used to diagnose constipation because stool was readily identified. However, the fever and the productive cough were due to pneumonia, which had to be treated immediately. The first clue was the cough, the respiratory rate of 24, and the bilateral crackles. The chest x-ray revealed a pleural effusion.

Imipenem and cilastatin (Primaxin) was ordered. The usual dose is 250–500 mg IV every 6 hours. Because of the patient's renal history and age, the dose was decreased to 500 mg every 12 hours after consultation with the pharmacy. This medication can only be administered by IV or IM. The patient and his daughter were instructed on his medications. During the hospital admission, further assessment was conducted on his renal status, BPH, and noted tremors.

Case Study Inquiry

16

Vocabulary

Self-Query

Before attempting to work the case study, define each of the vocabulary words. Although the words may have several subheadings, it will give you a place to begin your inquiry.

Alveoli
_____

Atelectasis
_____

Community-acquired pneumonia
_____

Herpes zoster infection (shingles)
_____

Hospital-acquired pneumonia
_____

Lung abscess
_____

Pericarditis
_____

Pleural effusion
_____

Pleurisy
_____

Severe acute respiratory syndrome (SARS)
_____

Ventilator-acquired pneumonia
_____

You are assessing a new home health patient. She is 82 years of age and in fairly good health. She has recently been discharged from the hospital. She was admitted for repair of a hip fracture to the right femoral head and developed pneumonia while there. She was also diagnosed with pernicious anemia. She will be seen by the nurses and physical therapist.

Home Medications Before Hospital Admission

Aspirin (ASA) 81 mg daily orally

Calcium citrate (Citracal) with vitamin D 2 tabs 3 times a day

Furosemide (Lasix) 40 mg daily orally

Omega-3 two tabs with breakfast

Potassium chloride 20 mEq daily orally

᪥ Self-Query

Using a drug book or pharmacology text that contains the mechanism of action, unlabeled uses, and pharmacokinetics for medications, answer the following questions. Make answers specific to this scenario.

What do I know about these medications? Do I know the recommended dose of, the recommended route for, and the best time of day to give these medications? Do I know what lab results I need regarding each medication? Do I know the approved use of each medication? Do I know the most common diseases treated by the listed medications? Are any off-label uses approved for each drug?

Aspirin

_____

_____

Calcium citrate with vitamin D

_____

_____

Furosemide

_____

_____

Omega-3

_____

_____

Potassium chloride

_____

_____

Can I list the individual's past medical history by looking at the medication list?

_____

_____

Home Medications After Hospital Discharge

Aspirin 81 mg daily orally

Azithromycin 250 mg twice a day before meals

Calcium citrate with vitamin D 2 tabs 3 times a day

Cyanocobalamin (Vitamin B12) 1000 mcg/mL IM monthly

Furosemide 40 mg daily orally

Omega-3 two tabs with breakfast

Potassium chloride 20 mEq daily orally

᪥ Self-Query

What was the most likely causative agent for the patient's pneumonia?

_____

_____

The patient's grandson, who is in the room, makes a remark that several months ago he also took azithromycin for his stomach ulcer along with several other medications. Is this likely? If so, what most likely caused the grandson's stomach ulcer?

_____

_____

The patient wants to know why she cannot take a pill for her anemia. She does not really want a "shot" every month. Explain the reason for the injection.

_____

_____

Nursing Process

Self-Query

What nursing assessment will I perform regarding each medication? What planning and implementation do I need to conduct for each medication? How do I evaluate each medication's effectiveness?

Aspirin

_____

_____

Azithromycin

_____

_____

Calcium citrate with vitamin D

_____

_____

Cyanocobalamin

_____

_____

Furosemide

_____

_____

Omega-3

_____

_____

Potassium chloride

_____

_____

Do I need to be concerned about geriatric considerations with this individual?

_____

_____

Synopsis

16

Because you can find answers to the self-queries in numerous texts, you will not find the answers to all of them here. However, you will find discussion of the individual case. The scenario relates to a geriatric individual with a history of hip replacement. She developed pneumonia while in the hospital and was also diagnosed with pernicious anemia. Therefore, purposefully look into the medication use and vocabulary as they relate to these factors.

Vocabulary

When reviewing the vocabulary words, you might want to ask several questions: who, what, where, when, why, and how. This should give you a much broader understanding of each word.

Do yourself a favor and do not just give the shortest and simplest answer. Use the following example of atelectasis: Instead of answering, "Atelectasis is another term for the alveoli being collapsed," ask:

Why did this woman develop **atelectasis**? Who is at risk for atelectasis? What medications can cause atelectasis? What treatments are used to prevent atelectasis?

☑ Self-Query: Possible Answers

When defining the remainder of the vocabulary words, ask the following questions:

Where are **alveoli** located? Why are they needed?

Who is at risk for **community-acquired pneumonia (CAP)**? What are the treatments for CAP? How can CAP be prevented?

Who is at risk for **herpes zoster infection (shingles)**? What is the treatment for shingles? How can shingles be prevented in the geriatric population?

Why did this woman develop **hospital-acquired pneumonia (HAP)**? Who is at risk for HAP? What are the treatments for HAP? How can it be prevented?

What is a **lung abscess**? Who is at risk for developing a lung abscess?

Who is at risk for **pericarditis**? What treatments are used to prevent pericarditis?

Which medications may actually cause pericarditis?

Why did this woman develop a **pleural effusion**? Who is at risk for pleural effusion? Where are most pleural effusions located? What treatments are used to prevent pleural effusions?

Who is at risk for **pleurisy**? What treatments are used to prevent pleurisy?

Who is at risk for **severe acute respiratory syndrome (SARS)**? What is the treatment for SARS? How can SARS be prevented?

Who is at risk for **ventilator-acquired pneumonia (VAP)**? What are the treatments for VAP? How can VAP be prevented?

Home Medications After Hospital Discharge

☑ Self-Query: Possible Answers

Most of the prehospital medications reveal a cardiac history. Before the patient's hip surgery, she was cleared by her cardiac physician; the blood work revealed decreased RBCs and platelets. A loss of coordination was also a clue and precipitated her fall and subsequent hip fracture.

She developed symptoms 72 hours after her surgery. It was hospital acquired. Her initial chest X-ray, taken by her cardiologist to clear her for surgery, was clear. The most common pathogens are gram-negative bacilli and *Staphylococcus aureus*.

She was placed on azithromycin 250 mg every 12 hours. Her grandson stated he also had been prescribed azithromycin (which he knew as Zithromax). He was taking the medication for *Helicobacter pylori* eradication, the causative factor of his duodenal ulcer.

Teaching needs to be done concerning the need for the B12 as an injection.

You will need to explain the connection between intrinsic factors and the absorption of B12. Explain why it must be given by IM and not by mouth. How is the intrinsic factor affected in individuals in this patient's age group?

Case Study Inquiry

17

Vocabulary

Self-Query

Before attempting to work the case study, define each of the vocabulary words. Although the words may have several subheadings, it will give you a place to begin your inquiry.

Antinuclear antibody (ANA)

_____

Autoimmune disease

_____

Connective tissue disease

_____

Disease-modifying antirheumatic drug (DMARD)

_____

Erythrocyte sedimentation rate (ESR)

_____

Nonsteroidal anti-inflammatory drug (NSAID)

_____

Osteoarthritis (OA)

_____

Rheumatoid arthritis (RA)

_____

Serum complement

_____

Synovitis

_____

You are assessing a new admission to your orthopedic floor. She is 29 years of age and is to undergo a synovectomy. She arrives in a wheelchair and needs additional assistance to walk to the bed. Her children, 6 and 8 years of age, are present. She has her lab work from the previous day and a list of her medications. She is 5'7" and weighs 125 pounds. She is having the surgery before her youngest child begins school; she is hoping that she can at least be a homeroom helper at her children's school.

Home Medications

Docusate/sennosides (Senokot-S) 2 tabs every 8 hours
Methotrexate 20 mg orally every Monday
Morphine (MSIR) 10 mg orally as needed for breakthrough pain
Morphine sulfate controlled-release (MS Contin) 30 mg orally every 12 hours
Prednisone 5 mg orally

Using a drug book or pharmacology text that contains the mechanism of action, unlabeled uses, and pharmacokinetics for medications, answer the following questions. Make answers specific to this scenario.

Do I know why the patient is taking these medications? What do I know about these medications? For each medication, what is the recommended dose, recommended route, and best time of day to give it? Do I know what lab results I need in regard to each medication? Do I know the approved use of each medication? Do I know the most common diseases treated by the listed medications? Are any off-label uses approved for each drug?

Docusate/sennosides

_____

_____

Methotrexate

_____

_____

Morphine

_____

_____

Morphine sulfate controlled-release

_____

_____

Prednisone

_____

_____

Do I know the different uses for methotrexate?

_____

Do I know why methotrexate is only given once a week and not daily?

_____

Discharge Medications

The procedure is a success, and the patient is discharged home with physical therapy.

Docusate/sennosides 2 tabs every 8 hours

Etanercept (Enbrel) 0.08 mg/kg subcutaneously once weekly

Methotrexate 20 mg orally every Monday

Morphine IR 10 mg orally as needed for breakthrough pain

Morphine sulfate controlled-release 30 mg orally every 12 hours

Self-Query

What has been added and why?

_____

_____

What has been removed and why?

_____

_____

What is the classification of etanercept (Enbrel)?

_____

_____

Write a teaching plan for patient and family education.

_____

_____

_____

Calculate the patient's dose of etanercept before she leaves.

_____

What is the yearly cost of this patient's medications?

_____

Follow-up

The patient has been taking her medications and doing better, and she has been assisting her child's teacher at school. Three of her daughter's friends are absent from school on Friday. Late on Monday, the patient develops red raised vesicular lesions on her face and trunk. On Tuesday, she has a fever of 101.2°F and severe fatigue. The teacher calls her and tells her to remain at home because several children have chickenpox. The patient calls her physician and is told to report to the hospital immediately. She is now 5'7" and 120 pounds.

Physician Orders

Stop methotrexate 20 mg orally every Monday

Stop etanercept 0.08 mg/kg subcutaneously once weekly

Start acyclovir 15 mg/kg/daily; divide over 8 hours

Chest X-ray, monitor oxygen saturation every 4 hours

Place patient in strict isolation (no visitors); obtain a creatinine clearance before acyclovir

Self-Query

Why do you think these two medications have been discontinued?

_____

_____

What are the classifications of the discontinued medications?

_____

What do you need to obtain for the pharmacy to calculate her dose of acyclovir? After obtaining information from the pharmacy, what other information is necessary?

_____

_____

Why has the dose been ordered this way?

_____

_____

How should you administer the acyclovir?

_____

_____

What is a toxic effect if acyclovir if it is administered too quickly?

_____

_____

The patient recovers after 7 days of IV acyclovir therapy and is discharged home.

Home Medications

Morphine sulfate controlled-release 30 mg orally every 12 hours

Morphine 10 mg orally as needed for breakthrough pain

Senokot-S 2 tabs every 8 hours

Acyclovir 200 mg orally 3 times a day for 5 days

Stop methotrexate 20 mg orally every Monday until seen by the physician in 2 weeks

Stop etanercept 0.08 mg/kg subcutaneously once weekly until seen by the physician in 2 weeks

Nursing Process

Self-Query

The patient is now concerned about her medications and wonders why she continues to take acyclovir given that her rash is gone. What is your reply?

_____

_____

She wants to know why she cannot immediately restart the methotrexate and etanercept. What is your reply? How will your answer affect the way she takes her medications in the future?

_____

_____

_____

What lab results will need to be assessed regularly?

_____

_____

Reviewing the scenario, what do you think happened to the patient?

_____

_____

Synopsis

17

Because you can find answers to the self-queries in numerous texts, you will not find the answers to all of them here. However, you will find discussion of the individual case. The scenario relates to a 29-year-old with a rheumatoid disorder; therefore, purposefully look into the medication use and vocabulary as they relate to these factors.

Vocabulary

When reviewing the vocabulary words, you might want to ask several questions: who, what, where, when, why, and how. This should give you a much broader understanding of each word.

Do yourself a favor and do not just give the shortest and simplest answer. Use the following example of connective tissue disease: Instead of answering, "Connective tissue disease is any disease that targets the connective tissues of the body," ask:

Why did this patient develop a **connective tissue disease**? Who is at risk for connective tissue disease? What medications can cause connective tissue disease? What medications are used to prevent connective tissue disease?

☑ Self-Query: Possible Answers

When defining the remainder of the vocabulary words, ask the following questions:

What is an **antinuclear antibody (ANA)**? What does it detect? How is the test evaluated?

Why did this patient develop an **autoimmune disease**? Who is at risk for autoimmune diseases? What medications are used to treat autoimmune diseases?

What is a **disease-modifying antirheumatic drug (DMARD)**? Why is it used to treat connective tissue disease? Why is it used for RA? Is it used for OA?

What is an **erythrocyte sedimentation rate (ESR)**? What does it detect? How is the test evaluated?

What is **nonsteroidal anti-inflammatory drug (NSAID)**? Why is it used to treat connective tissue disease? Why is it used for RA? Why is it used for OA?

How is RA different from **osteoarthritis (OA)**? Who is at risk for OA? What medications are used to treat OA?

How did this patient develop **rheumatoid arthritis (RA)**? Who is at risk for RA? What medications are used to treat RA?

What is a **serum complement**? What does it detect? How is the test evaluated?

Why did this patient develop **synovitis**? Who is at risk for synovitis? What medications are used to treat synovitis?

Home Medications

✓ Self-Query: Possible Answers

Methotrexate (MTX) was originally used in cancer therapy. Methotrexate is commonly used to terminate early pregnancies, and now it is used as a treatment for certain autoimmune diseases.

Discharge Medications

✓ Self-Query: Possible Answers

The prednisone has been discontinued. We will focus on the addition of the etanercept (Enbrel) to the methotrexate. The treatment for this patient is referred to as evidence-based practice. Etanercept, a tumor necrosis factor blocker, has been shown to slow the progression of RA. The use of etanercept and methotrexate has shown even more promise.

Calculated dose 0.08 mg $\times$ 56.81 kg subcutaneously once a week

After the initial dose for 1 month, the physician increased the dose to 25 mg subcutaneously twice a week.

Nursing Process

✓ Self-Query: Possible Answers

Both of these medications have the risk of leaving the individual susceptible to serious infection.

The patient worked with children who developed chickenpox; normally, this would not have been so bad, but taking the medications for the RA decreased her immunity. This left her vulnerable to infections and severely immunocompromised. The physician was most concerned about the possibility of varicella pneumonia, a serious complication of varicella infection. This complication often results in respiratory failure and death. Dosage adjustment of acyclovir is recommended when administering to individuals with renal impairment. This is a possibility in this individual, considering all the other medications she has been prescribed for her RA. Better teaching is needed for this immunocompromised patient concerning the transmission of live viruses before she resumes her RA therapy of etanercept and methotrexate.

Case Study Inquiry

18

Vocabulary

⚲ Self-Query

Before attempting to work the case study, define each of the vocabulary words. Although the words may have several subheadings, it will give you a place to begin your inquiry.

Acetylcholine

_____

Anticholinergic agent

_____

Basal ganglion

_____

Bradykinesia

_____

Dopaminergic agents

_____

Extrapyramidal pathways

_____

Neurotransmitter

_____

Parkinson's disease (PD)

_____

A 71-year-old female is brought to the physician's office for a routine checkup. You are reviewing the following medications with her husband.

Home Medications

Aspirin and extended-release dipyridamole (Aggrenox) 25 mg/200 mg capsule twice a day orally
Carbidopa and levodopa (Parcopa) 25 mg/100 mg at 9 a.m., 5 p.m., and 11 p.m. orally
Docusate (Colace) 1 cap at bedtime
Furosemide 80 mg every morning orally
Latanoprost 1 drop left eye at bedtime
Metoprolol 12.5 mg once a day orally
Potassium chloride 20 mEq every day orally
Ranitidine (Zantac) 150 mg daily orally
Temazepam (Restoril) 7.5 mg with Parcopa

⚲ Self-Query

Using a drug book or pharmacology text that contains the mechanism of action, unlabeled uses, and pharmacokinetics for medications, answer the following questions. Make answers specific to this scenario.

What do I know about these medications? Do I know the recommended dose of, the recommended route for, and the best time of day to give these medications? Do I know what lab results I need regarding each medication? Do I know the approved use of each medication? Do I know the most common diseases treated by the listed medications? Are any off-label uses approved for each drug?

Aspirin and extended-release dipyridamole

_____

_____

Carbidopa and levodopa

_____

_____

Docusate

_____

_____

Furosemide

_____

_____

Latanoprost

_____

_____

Metoprolol

_____

_____

Potassium chloride

_____

_____

Ranitidine

_____

_____

Temazepam

_____

_____

Can I determine the individual's past medical history by looking at the medication list?

_____

Do I know possible drug interactions of medications on this list?

_____

Why is it important to assess the skin of anyone taking levodopa?

_____

Body Systems

Self-Query

Can I place each medication under the body system that it commonly affects?
Be prepared to defend your answers.

Neurological

_____

Cardiovascular

_____

Hematological

_____

Pulmonary

_____

Gastrointestinal

_____

Nutrition

_____

Genitourinary/renal

_____

Musculoskeletal

_____

Endocrine

_____

Integumentary

_____

Immune

_____

Pain/comfort

_____

Mechanism of Action

Self-Query

Am I aware of each medication's mechanism of action, and do I know possible drug interactions of medications on this list?

_____

_____

Does the individual's medical history have an effect on the pharmacokinetics of each drug?

_____

_____

What contraindications do I need to address regarding the medications and possible medical health history?

_____

_____

Nursing Process

Self-Query

What nursing assessment will I perform regarding each medication? What is a priority nursing diagnosis regarding each medication? What planning and implementation do I need to do in regard to each medication? How do I evaluate each medication's effectiveness?

Aspirin and extended-release dipyridamole

_____

_____

Carbidopa and levodopa

_____

_____

Docusate

_____

_____

Furosemide

_____

_____

Latanoprost

_____

_____

Metoprolol

_____

_____

Potassium chloride

_____

_____

Ranitidine

_____

_____

Temazepam

_____

_____

Do I need to be concerned about geriatric considerations with this individual?

_____

The patient asks why the doctor told her not to take diphenhydramine (Benadryl) for her allergies this spring. What can you tell her?

_____

_____

The patient also should not take metoclopramide (Reglan) for nausea. She wants to know why. What can you tell her?

_____

_____

What other medications are related to these two medications (diphenhydramine and metoclopramide)?

_____

_____

Synopsis

18

Because you can find answers to the self-queries in numerous texts, you will not find the answers to all of them here. However, you will find discussion of the individual case. The scenario relates to a 77-year-old female with Parkinson's disease; therefore, purposefully look into the medication use and vocabulary as they relate to these factors.

Vocabulary

When reviewing the vocabulary words, you might want to ask several questions: who, what, where, when, why, and how. This should give you a much broader understanding of each word.

Do yourself a favor and do not just give the shortest and simplest answer. Use the following example of Parkinson's disease: Instead of answering, "Parkinson's disease is a disease affecting the part of the brain associated with movement. It is characterized by shaking and difficulty with movement coordination," ask:

Why did this woman develop **Parkinson's disease (PD)**? Who is at risk for PD? What medications can cause symptoms of PD? What medications are used to decrease the symptoms of PD? What symptoms did this patient probably exhibit in the beginning?

☑ Self-Query: Possible Answers

When defining the remainder of the vocabulary words, ask the following questions:

What is **acetylcholine**? Where is it located? Why is it needed?

What is an **anticholinergic agent**? Why is one needed?

Where is the **basal ganglion**? How is it altered in PD patients?

What is **bradykinesia**? What medications can cause it? Who is at risk? How is it treated?

What are **dopaminergic agents**? Who needs them? How must they be delivered to be beneficial?

What is an **extrapyramidal pathway**? Where is it located? Why is it important? Which medications most alter this pathway?

What is a **neurotransmitter**? How many have been identified? Which medications most alter these transmitters? Where are they located? How are neurotransmitters altered in a patient with PD?

Home Medications

☑ Self-Query: Possible Answers

Consult any drug text that reads easily. Review the patient medications and list the possible past medical history.

Aspirin and extended-release dipyridamole (Aggrenox) capsules: Indicated to reduce the risk of stroke.

Carbidopa and levodopa (Parcopa): Parkinson's disease

Docusate (Colace): Self-medication for constipation

Furosemide: Hypertension, edema (possible heart failure)

Latanoprost: Glaucoma (open-angle type) or ocular hypertension

Metoprolol: Beta blocker—hypertension

Potassium chloride: Potassium supplement (taking due to also being on furosemide)

Ranitidine (Zantac): Self-medication for heartburn and indigestion

Temazepam: Insomnia

It is important to assess the skin of anyone taking levodopa because it may activate malignant melanoma, although research has yet to support anecdotal evidence that links levodopa and melanoma.

Body Systems

☑ Self-Query: Possible Answer

Neurological

> Carbidopa and levodopa
> Temazepam

Cardiac

> Furosemide
> Metoprolol
> Aspirin and extended-release dipyridamole

Hematological

> None

Pulmonary

> None

Gastrointestinal

> Ranitidine
> Docusate

Nutrition

> None

Genitourinary/renal

> Furosemide

Musculoskeletal

> None

Endocrine

> None

Integumentary

> None

Immune

    None

Pain/comfort

    Latanoprost (prostaglandin analog)

Nursing Process

☑ Self-Query: Possible Answers

The active medicine in diphenhydramine (Benadryl) was used before the availability of modern medications that treat the mild symptoms of PD. Because the patient is already on medication for PD, it is imperative that she not add to the effects of her present medication.

Metoclopramide (Reglan) is a dopamine receptor blocking agent and can cause symptoms of PD; it also worsens the already-present tremors related to PD. Remember that dopamine depletion is the problem in PD; therefore, metoclopramide should not be used in patients with diagnosed PD. She had requested it for her acid stomach, as she called it. She settled for ranitidine.

Case Study Inquiry

19

Vocabulary

🔎 Self-Query

Before attempting to work the case study, define each of the vocabulary words. Although the words may have several subheadings, it will give you a place to begin your inquiry.

Adrenal androgens

_____

Androgen dependent

_____

Brachytherapy

_____

Castration

_____

Digital rectal exam (DRE)

_____

Estrogen

_____

Prostate-specific antigen (PSA) level

_____

Testosterone

_____

A 75-year-old male is brought to the office for a checkup related to a diagnosis of prostatism. You are reviewing the following medications with the patient and his son.

Home Medications

Amlodipine (Norvasc) 2.5-mg tab once daily with breakfast

Aspirin (ASA) 325 mg orally as needed for joint pain

Ferrous gluconate 325-mg tab daily 1 hour before breakfast

Finasteride (Proscar) 5-mg tab daily orally

Naftifine topical cream 1% to affected area once daily; if no improvement return to physician's office for evaluation

Psyllium (Metamucil) 1 tsp every morning with orange juice

Tamsulosin (Flomax) 0.4 mg daily orally

Using a drug book or pharmacology text that contains the mechanism of action, unlabeled uses, and pharmacokinetics for medications, answer the following questions. Make answers specific to this scenario.

Why is the patient receiving each of the mediations? What do I know about these medications? Do I know the recommended dose of, the recommended route for, and the best time of day to give these medications? Do I know what lab results I need regarding each medication? Do I know the approved use of each medication? Do I know the most common diseases treated by the listed medications? Are any off-label uses approved for each drug?

Amlodipine

_____

_____

Aspirin

_____

_____

Ferrous gluconate

_____

_____

Finasteride

_____

_____

Naftifine topical cream

_____

_____

Psyllium

_____

_____

Tamsulosin

_____

_____

The patient states that amlodipine is a new drug for him, and he has an appointment to have the dosage adjusted every 2 weeks. Is this common with this medication? How is the dosage adjusted?

_____

_____

Nursing Process

? Self-Query

What nursing assessment will I perform regarding each medication? What planning and implementation do I need to do in regard to each medication? How do I evaluate each medication's effectiveness?

Amlodipine

_____

_____

Aspirin

_____

_____

Ferrous gluconate

_____

_____

Finasteride

_____

_____

Naftifine topical cream

_____

_____

Psyllium

_____

_____

Tamsulosin

_____

_____

Geriatric considerations: Are these medications for age-related diseases? Explain your answer.

_____

_____

The patient and his son have a few questions for you. First, they ask if he still needs to take his "prostate cancer drugs." Explain your answer.

_____

Next, they ask if he is receiving any cancer drugs. Explain your answer.

_____

_____

Develop a teaching plan for this patient concerning the use of finasteride and the tamsulosin, and explain why they are given.

_____

_____

_____

The patient also asks why the physician stopped his doxazosin (Cardura) and placed him on a different blood pressure drug. Is there a connection between doxazosin's classification and another medication that he is taking?

_____

_____

The patient mentions that a good friend told him about a drug called saw palmetto, and he wants to try it. What is saw palmetto? What does research data reveal about the product? How is it classified? What is its mechanism of action? Are there any adverse effects? Will it interact with any of his other medications? What will you tell the patient?

_____

_____

_____

Body Systems

⚲ Self-Query

Be prepared to defend your answers.

Can I place each medication under the body system that it commonly affects?

Neurological
_____

Cardiovascular
_____

Hematological
_____

Pulmonary
_____

Gastrointestinal
_____

Nutrition
_____

Genitourinary/renal
_____

Musculoskeletal
_____

Endocrine
_____

Integumentary
_____

Immune
_____

Pain/comfort
_____

Synopsis

19

Because you can find answers to the self-queries in numerous texts, you will not find the answers to all of them here. However, you will find discussion of the individual case. The scenario relates to a 75-year-old male with a history of prostate problems. He is in the office for a routine visit. Therefore, purposefully look into the medication use and vocabulary as they relate to this situation.

Vocabulary

When reviewing the vocabulary words, you might want to ask several questions: who, what, where, when, why, and how. This should give you a much broader understanding of each word.

Do yourself a favor and do not just give the shortest and simplest answer. Use the following example of androgen-dependent diseases: Instead of answering, "Androgen dependent relates to any group of hormones that influence the male reproductive system," ask:

What are the **androgen-dependent** diseases? What conditions are androgen dependent? Are there any androgen independent diseases? How are the treatments different?

☑ Self-Query: Possible Answers

When defining the remainder of the vocabulary words, ask the following questions:

What are **adrenal androgens**? Why are they important? Who needs them? What role do they play in prostate cancer? Where are they produced?

What is **brachytherapy**? How is it used to treat prostate and other cancers? What are the different types of brachytherapy? What are some of the major side effects of brachytherapy?

What is **castration**? What is pharmacologic castration? What are the uses for castration? How is it a treatment for prostate cancer?

What is a **digital rectal exam (DRE)**? Why is it important? What does it measure? What role does it play in prostate cancer? What exactly does it examine? How is it performed?

What is **estrogen**? Why is estrogen important? Who needs it? What role does it play in prostate cancer? Where is it produced?

What is a **prostate-specific antigen (PSA) level**? Why is it important? What does it measure? What role does it play in prostate cancer? Where is it produced?

What is **testosterone**? Why is it important? Who needs it? What role does it play in prostate cancer? Where is it produced?

Home Medications

☑ Self-Query: Possible Answers

Having the dosage adjusted every 2 weeks is common with amlodipine (Norvasc). Also, the patient should be instructed to avoid drinking grapefruit juice with the medication.

Nursing Process

☑ Self-Query: Possible Answers

Finasteride (Proscar) is used in the treatment of symptomatic benign prostatic hyperplasia (BPH). Tamsulosin (Flomax) is an alpha-1 blocker used in the reduction of BPH.

The patient's doxazosin (Cardura) was stopped because it is an alpha adrenergic blocker; it cannot be used in conjunction with tamsulosin.

Saw palmetto is used in alternative medicine to aid in the treatment of BPH. Research of high methodological quality has indicated no difference from placebo in treating BPH. A healthcare provider should be consulted regarding the use of this and any other alternative medication.

Naftifine is an antifungal medication; this patient was diagnosed with ringworm.

Body Systems

☑ Self-Query: Possible Answers

Neurological

　None

Cardiovascular

　Amlodipine

Hematological

　Ferrous gluconate

Pulmonary

　None

Gastrointestinal

　Psyllium

Nutrition

　None

Genitourinary/renal

　Tamsulosin

Musculoskeletal

　Aspirin

Endocrine

　None

Integumentary

　Naftifine

Immune

　None

Pain/comfort

　Aspirin

Case Study Inquiry

20

Vocabulary

Self-Query

Before attempting to work the case study, define the vocabulary words. Although the words may have several subheadings, it will give you a place to begin your inquiry.

Angina

_____

Anticoagulant

_____

Antiplatelet

_____

C-reactive protein

_____

Echocardiogram

_____

Homocysteine

_____

Pericarditis

_____

Polypharmacy

_____

Transesophageal echocardiogram (TEE)

_____

You are attempting to do medication reconciliation for an individual brought into the emergency department by ambulance. The patient, an 85-year-old female, called the ambulance when she began vomiting. Over the past few days, she has become extremely fatigued when retrieving her mail at the front door. She has a history of cardiac disease that appeared mostly after suffering an anterior myocardial infarction 5 years ago. She was recently classified as a New York Heart Association Class III (NYHA III). She was discharged 1 week ago following treatment for a UTI, and she had cataract surgery 2 days ago.

Emergency Department Assessment

The patient is weak and cannot walk 8 feet without severe dyspneic episodes. She also noted urinary incontinence during ambulation. She states that she has a "really bad headache" and feels a little "shaky." She states that she took all her medications this morning but did not feel like eating afterward.

She states that she placed a heart pill under her tongue when she started vomiting. She does not report severe thirst, and she denies chest pain. She presents you with a list of her medications.

Self-Query

Do I have an idea of what the "heart pill" is?

Home Medications

Aspirin (ASA) 324 mg for arthritis pain every morning at 8 a.m.

Atenolol (Tenormin) 25 mg 1 tab every day

Bismuth subsalicylate (Pepto-Bismol) daily for upset stomach

Calcium citrate (Citracal) 250 mg with vitamin D, 2 tabs daily with meals

Carvedilol (Coreg) 6.25-mg tab every morning before breakfast and at 6 p.m.

Clopidogrel (Plavix) 75 mg daily at 6 p.m.

Furosemide (Lasix) 40 mg every morning at 8 a.m.

Furosemide 20 mg 2 tabs every morning with breakfast

Irbesartan (Avapro) 150 mg every afternoon after lunch

Levothyroxine (Synthroid) 112 mcg every morning at 8 a.m.

Metformin (Glucophage) 500 mg orally every morning with breakfast and again at 6 p.m.

Metformin 500 mg every morning with breakfast

Moxifloxacin (Vigamox) 1 drop to left eye every morning until post-op office visit

Multivitamin with iron (Icaps) 20 mEq daily, take with vitamin E

Pioglitazone (Actos) 15 mg every morning at 8 a.m.

Potassium chloride (K-Dur) 20-mEq tab orally at 6 p.m.

Psyllium (Metamucil) 1 tablespoon mixed with water every morning

Simvastatin (Zocor) 40 mg orally with evening medications

Vitamin E 1 tab of 400 units every morning with moxifloxacin

You see that the list is dated 2 days ago and ask who wrote it. The patient states that a neighbor came over and wrote down all the medications that were in her medicine cabinet so that her daughter could set them up for her to take. The neighbor wanted to be helpful because the patient had had eye surgery and could not see very well. The patient asks if there is something wrong with the list.

Self-Query

Using a drug book or pharmacology text that contains the mechanism of action, unlabeled uses, and pharmacokinetics for medications, answer the following questions. Make answers specific to this scenario.

What do I know about these medications? Do I know the recommended dose of, the recommended route for, and the best time of day to give these medications? Do I know what lab results I need regarding each medication? Do I know the approved use of each medication? Do I know the most common diseases treated by the listed medications? Are any off-label uses approved for each drug?

Aspirin

_____

_____

Atenolol

_____

_____

Bismuth subsalicylate

_____

_____

Calcium citrate

_____

_____

Carvedilol

_____

_____

Clopidogrel

_____

_____

Furosemide

_____

_____

Irbesartan

_____

_____

Levothyroxine

_____

_____

Metformin

_____

_____

Moxifloxacin

_____

_____

Multivitamin with iron

_____

_____

Pioglitazone

_____

_____

Potassium chloride

_____

_____

Psyllium

_____

_____

Simvastatin

_____

_____

Vitamin E

_____

_____

Do I see anything immediately "wrong" with the list? If so, what?

_____

Were any of the dosages copied incorrectly?

_____

What mistake did the neighbor make? How could it have been avoided?

_____

_____

Are all the listed home medications necessary?

_____

_____

Looking at the list of medications, what medical history do I expect to find other than what the patient has stated?

_____

_____

Body Systems

Self-Query

Be prepared to defend your answers.

Can I place each medication under the body system that it commonly affects?

Neurological

_____

Cardiovascular

_____

Hematological

_____

Pulmonary

_____

Gastrointestinal

_____

Nutrition

_____

Genitourinary/renal

_____

Musculoskeletal

_____

Endocrine

_____

Integumentary

_____

Immune

_____

Pain/comfort

_____

Mechanism of Action

Self-Query

Does the individual's medical history have an effect on the pharmacokinetics of each drug?

_____

_____

What contraindications do I need to address regarding the medications and medical history?

_____

_____

Nursing Process

Self-Query

What nursing assessment do I need to perform regarding each medication? What is a priority nursing diagnosis regarding each medication? What planning and implementation do I need to do for each medication? How do I evaluate each medication's effectiveness?

Aspirin

_____

_____

Atenolol

_____

_____

Bismuth subsalicylate

_____

_____

Calcium citrate

_____

_____

Carvedilol

_____

_____

Clopidogrel

_____

_____

Furosemide

_____

_____

Irbesartan

_____

_____

Levothyroxine

_____

_____

Metformin

_____

_____

Moxifloxacin

_____

_____

Multivitamin with iron

_____

_____

Pioglitazone

_____

_____

Potassium chloride

_____

_____

Psyllium

_____

_____

Simvastatin

_____

_____

Vitamin E

_____

_____

Physical Assessment Findings

Blood pressure 90/50

Heart rate 118

Temperature 100.2°F

Potassium 2.5

Blood glucose 55

Sodium 128

Physician Orders

Stop all home meds until further assessment.

NS at 100 mL/hr

Add 40 mEg KCL to each bag of 1000 mL NS

Give 1/2 amp of dextrose 50 and redraw blood glucose in 2 hours

Lab orders: Salicylate level, BUN, creatinine, PT/INR, T_3 and T_4 levels, calcium levels

Self-Query

What type of solution is NS?

_____

Why not use dextrose as the infusion therapy?

_____

What will the 1/2 amp of dextrose 50 accomplish?

_____

Look at the lab orders. Which lab orders match up with which medications?

_____

_____

_____

Nursing Process

After 3 days in the hospital, the patient has recovered and is being discharged.

Self-Query

What teaching should be done so that this scenario does not happen again?

_____

_____

What should be done with medications that she no longer takes?

_____

Synopsis

20

Because you can find answers to the self-queries in numerous texts, you will not find the answers to all of them here. However, you will find discussion of the individual case. The scenario relates to a 85-year-old female with a history of cardiac problems. The issues presently relate to polypharmacy. Therefore, purposefully look into the medication use and vocabulary as they relate to these factors.

Vocabulary

When reviewing the vocabulary words, you might want to ask several questions: who, what, where, when, why, and how. This should give you a much broader understanding of each word.

Do yourself a favor and do not just give the shortest and simplest answer. Use the following example of antiplatelet: Instead of answering, "An antiplatelet is anything that interferes with the blood's ability to clot," ask:

What medications are classified as **antiplatelets**? Why was this individual prescribed an antiplatelet? How can aspirin be an antiplatelet, an antipyretic, and an anti-inflammatory?

☑ Self-Query: Possible Answers

When defining the remainder of all vocabulary words, ask the following questions:

What is **angina**? How are antiplatelet medications used in the treatment of angina? How are anticoagulation medications used in the treatment of angina?

What medications are classified as **anticoagulants**? Are antiplatelet medications different from anticoagulate medications? Who uses anticoagulation medications? What is the difference between an antiplatelet and an anticoagulant?

What is **C-reactive protein**? What is its role in heart disease? How is it measured?

What is an **echocardiogram**? How is it performed? Who has it performed? What would you expect to find in a person with an NYHA III classification?

What is **homocysteine**? What is its role in heart disease? Where is it located?

What is **pericarditis**? How is it caused? Who is at risk? Would you expect to find pericarditis in this individual?

What is **polypharmacy**? Who is most likely to have this issue?

What is a **transesophageal echocardiogram** (TEE)? How is it performed? Who has it performed? What would you expect to find in a person with an NYHA III classification?

Home Medications

☑ Self-Query: Possible Answers

How this unfolded: This individual has numerous ailments and keeps all her medications, including those that she should have discarded. Her neighbor was not aware of this. When the neighbor came to help, she was not aware that the patient did not actually take all the medications in the cabinet, and she wrote them all down.

So, for at least 24 hours, the patient has been taking all her medications, past and present. The patient's daughter, who lives with her and assists in giving her the medications, is 65 years old and also in poor health. No one was around to question the numerous medications; this situation emphasizes the importance of teaching and giving instructions regarding all medications and their handling. Medications are expensive; however, they should always be discarded when discontinued.

The pill that the patient took was sublingual nitroglycerine. We need to see what is on the list and then collaborate with the physician and the pharmacist to see what the patient should be taking. Combining the medications, we see the following medications with the same classifications:

Antidiabetics

Pioglitazone (Actos) 15 mg every morning at 8
The following are the same medications:
Metformin (Glucophage) 500 mg orally every morning with breakfast and again at 6 p.m.
Metformin 500 mg every morning with breakfast

Antihypertensives

Irbesartan (Avapro) 150 mg every afternoon after lunch
Carvedilol (Coreg) 6.25-mg tab every morning before breakfast and at 6 p.m.
Atenolol (Tenormin) 25 mg 1 tab every day

Antiplatelets

Aspirin (ASA) 324 mg for arthritis pain every morning at 8 a.m.
Clopidogrel (Plavix) 75 mg daily at 6 p.m.

Antihyperlipidemics

Simvastatin (Zocor) 40 mg orally with evening medications

Electrolyte replacements

Potassium chloride (K-Dur) 20-mEq tab orally at 6 p.m.

Diuretics

Furosemide (Lasix) 40 mg every morning at 8 a.m.
Furosemide 20 mg 2 tabs every morning with breakfast

Thyroid hormone replacements

Levothyroxine (Synthroid) 112 mcg every morning at 8 a.m.

Since the date of cataract surgery

Moxifloxacin (Vigamox) 1 drop to left eye every morning until postop office visit
Vitamin E 1 tab of 400 units every morning with moxifloxacin
Multivitamin with iron (Icaps) 20 mEq daily with vitamin E
Calcium citrate (Citracal) 250 mg with vitamin D, 2 tabs daily with meals

Over-the-counter self-medication for gastric distress

Bismuth subsalicylate (Pepto-Bismol) daily for upset stomach

Over-the-counter self-medication for constipation

Psyllium (Metamucil) 1 tbsp mixed with water every morning

Body Systems

☑ Self-Query: Possible Answers

Neurological

> None; however, the use of medications such as the diabetic medications will definitely affect her mental status.

Cardiovascular

> Irbesartan 150 mg every afternoon after lunch
> Carvedilol 6.25-mg tab every morning before breakfast and at 6 p.m.
> Atenolol 25 mg 1 tab every day
> Aspirin 324 mg for arthritis pain every morning at 8 a.m.
> Clopidogrel 75 mg daily at 6 p.m.
> Antihyperlipidemic
> Simvastatin 40 mg orally with evening medications

Hematological

> Aspirin 324 mg for arthritis pain every morning at 8 a.m.
> Clopidogrel 75 mg daily at 6 p.m.

Pulmonary

> None

Gastrointestinal

> Bismuth subsalicylate daily for upset stomach
> Psyllium 1 tbsp mixed with water every morning

Nutrition
> None

Genitourinary/renal

> Furosemide 40 mg every morning at 8 a.m.
> Furosemide 20 mg 2 tabs every morning with breakfast

Musculoskeletal

> Aspirin 324 mg for arthritis pain every morning at 8 a.m.
> Calcium citrate 250 mg with vitamin D, 2 tabs daily with meals

Endocrine

> Levothyroxine 112 mcg every morning at 8 a.m.

Integumentary

> None

Immune

> None

Pain/comfort

> Aspirin 324 mg for arthritis pain every morning at 8 a.m.

Physician Orders

☑ Self-Query: Possible Answers

The patient was dehydrated (as was reflected in the patient's blood pressure, heart rate, and temperature). However, she did not detect thirst; possibly because of her age, her *thirst* mechanisms and sensitivity were compromised.

Her heart rate, although elevated, was somewhat blunted because of the beta blocker she received. The potassium of 2.5 leads us to believe that she was taking both furosemide prescriptions. The glucose level was also low, leading us to believe that continuing on this route would have led to a dangerous level of hypoglycemia for the patient. The low sodium also may have led to the patient's confusion, and she was placed on seizure precautions. Renal studies were performed to assess for hypoperfusion; it was minimal.

The individual was discharged to an assisted living facility with the following medications:

Carvedilol 6.25-mg tab every morning before breakfast and at 6 p.m.
Atenolol 25 mg 1 tab every day
Aspirin 324 mg for arthritis pain every morning at 8 a.m.
Simvastatin 40 mg orally with evening medications
Potassium chloride 20-mEq tab orally at 6 p.m.
Furosemide 40 mg 2 tabs every morning with breakfast
Levothyroxine 112 mcg every morning at 8 a.m.
Moxifloxacin 1 drop to left eye every morning until postop office visit
Vitamin E 1 tab of 400 units every morning with moxifloxacin
Multivitamin with iron 20 mEq daily taken with vitamin E
Calcium citrate 250 mg with vitamin D, 2 tabs daily with meals

The patient was instructed to call the healthcare provider if she developed constipation. She was also instructed to check her blood sugar every other day and call for an appointment if it remained over 150 for 2 days. The patient and her daughter will continue to live together.

Case Study Inquiry

21

Vocabulary

Self-Query

Before attempting to work the case study, define the vocabulary words. Although the words may have several subheadings, it will give you a place to begin your inquiry.

Apraxia
_____

Cognition
_____

Confabulation
_____

Delirium
_____

Dementia
_____

Genetics
_____

Mini-mental state exam (MMSE)
_____

Wandering
_____

The patient is a 66-year-old female brought to the clinic because of repeated episodes of falling. Her husband has also noticed an increase in irritability over the past few weeks. He cannot quite put his finger on the problem, but he knows that something is wrong. After the fall this morning, he insisted on bringing in his wife for a checkup. He states that he has also noticed weight loss over the past month. The patient says that everyone can stand to lose a little weight.

Home Medications

Acetaminophen and diphenhydramine (Tylenol PM) 1 tab at bedtime
Albuterol (90 mcg) 2 puffs every 4 hours as needed
Alprazolam 0.25 mg orally 3 times a day with meals
Aspirin (ASA) 81 mg with breakfast
Bumetanide (Bumex) 1 mg orally daily
Clopidogrel 75 mg orally daily
Diphenhydramine (Benadryl) 25 mg orally at bedtime
Enalapril (Vasotec) 5 mg orally every 12 hours
Omeprazole 20 mg orally daily
Temazepam 50 mg at bedtime

Self-Query

Using a drug book or pharmacology text that contains the mechanism of action, unlabeled uses, and pharmacokinetics for medications, answer the following questions. Make answers specific to this scenario.

What do I know about these medications? Do I know the recommended dose of, the recommended route for, and the best time of day to give these medications? Do I know what lab results I need regarding each medication? Do I know the approved use of each medication? Do I know the most common diseases treated by the listed medications? Are any off-label uses approved for each drug?

Acetaminophen and diphenhydramine

_____

_____

Albuterol

_____

_____

Alprazolam

_____

_____

Aspirin

_____

_____

Bumetanide

_____

_____

Clopidogrel

_____

_____

Diphenhydramine

_____

_____

Enalapril

_____

_____

Omeprazole

_____

_____

Temazepam

_____

_____

Do I know the individual's past medical history by looking at the medication list?

_____

_____

Physician Orders I

After speaking with the patient and her husband, the physician decides to stop the following medications:

Temazepam 50 mg at bedtime

Clopidogrel 75 mg orally daily

Acetaminophen and diphenhydramine 1 capsule at bedtime (changed to plain acetominophen [Tylenol])

Diphenhydramine 25 mg orally at bedtime

Self-Query

Do I know why the physician would stop these medications?

_____

_____

Is the patient possibly taking duplicate medications?

_____

Follow-up I

A follow-up visit is scheduled, and the patient and her husband return to the clinic. She has not fallen since the last visit; however, she seems to be more depressed. Recently, she went shopping with her daughter and forgot her purse and house keys. She is admitted to your neurological unit for evaluation.

Physician Orders II

PET scan, electrolytes, B12 level, folate levels, thyroid and liver function test, serology for syphilis, BUN, creatinine, CBC, chemistry panel

Perform the MMSE

Assessment Findings

Lab results within the normal range for age

PET scan reveals decreased metabolic activity

MMSE score of 30

With these findings, the physician prescribes two new medications for discharge:

Memantine (Namenda) 10 mg until next office visit in 1 week

Donepezil (Aricept) 5 mg orally at bedtime until next office visit in 1 week

What are the most likely diagnosis and the prognosis for this patient?

_____

_____

What do I know about these medications? Do I know the recommended dose of, the recommended route for, and the best time of day to give these medications? Do I know what lab results I need regarding each medication? Do I know the approved use of each medication? Do I know the most common diseases treated by the listed medications? Are any off-label uses approved for each drug?

Memantine

_____

_____

Donepezil

_____

_____

What has research shown about the combination of these two medications?

_____

_____

Follow-up II

⁇ Self-Query

Answer the following questions, posed by the patient's son and daughter at the next office visit.

Does vitamin E slow the effects of the diagnosis?

_____

Do NSAIDs help slow the progression?

_____

Does ginkgo biloba show any results, and is it ever used?

_____

What are the benefits of the two new medications? How long before the family sees improvement? What side effects should they report? What should they do for major side effects? What should the family do if the patient misses a dose?

Memantine

_____

_____

Donepezil

_____

_____

Present Home Medications

Acetominophen 1 tab at bedtime

Albuterol (90 mcg) 2 puffs every 4 hours as needed

Aspirin 81 mg with breakfast

Bumetanide 1 mg orally daily

Donepezil 5 mg orally at bedtime until next office visit in 1 week

Enalapril 5 mg orally every 12 hours

Memantine 10 mg until next office visit in 1 week

Omeprazole 20 mg orally daily

Nursing Process

Self-Query

What nursing assessment will I perform for each medication? What planning and implementation do I need to do in regard to each medication? How do I evaluate each medication's effectiveness?

Acetominophen

_____

_____

Albuterol

_____

_____

Aspirin

_____

_____

Bumetanide

_____

_____

Donepezil

_____

_____

Enalapril

_____

_____

Memantine

_____

_____

Omeprazole

_____

_____

Is there a special diet for this patient?

_____

Is Alzheimer's an age-related disease? Explain your answer.

_____

_____

Synopsis

21

Because you can find answers to the self-queries in numerous texts, you will not find the answers to all of them here. However, you will find discussion of the individual case. The scenario relates to a 66-year-old female with a history of mental status changes; therefore, purposefully look into the medication use and vocabulary as they relate to these factors.

Vocabulary

When reviewing the vocabulary words, you might want to ask several questions: who, what, where, when, why, and how. This should give you a much broader understanding of each word.

Do yourself a favor and do not just give the shortest and simplest answer. The following questions are to be used as a guide. Apply the following mini-mental state exam (MMSE) example to all the vocabulary words. Instead of answering, "The MMSE is a set of questions that provides a score regarding a person's general level of mental ability," ask:

How is the **mini-mental state exam (MMSE)** used? Why is it used in cases of suspected Alzheimer's disease? What are the components of the exam?

☑ Self-Query: Possible Answers

When defining the remainder of the vocabulary words, ask the following questions:

What is **apraxia**? Who is at risk for apraxia? Which body system is altered in apraxia?

What is **cognition**? How is it altered? Who is at risk for altered cognition?

What is **confabulation**? How is it caused? What does it indicate?

What is **delirium**? Who is at risk for delirium?

What is **dementia**? How is it caused? Who is at risk? Would you expect to find dementia in this individual?

What is **genetics**? How is Alzheimer's genetically linked?

What is **wandering**? What causes it? Who is at risk for wandering?

Home Medications

☑ Self-Query: Possible Answers

Albuterol—pulmonary
Alprazolam—anxiety
Bumetanide (Bumex)—edema
Enalapril (Vasotec)—hypertension
Omeprazole—gastric reflux
Temazepam 50—insomnia
Aspirin (ASA)—cardiovascular
Acetaminophen and diphenhydramine (Tylenol PM), diphenhydramine (Benadryl)—pain and insomnia

Assessment Findings

☑ Self-Query: Possible Answers

Medications were discontinued if the individual was taking a duplicate medication. Although the MMSE was normal, the PET scan was more predictive of the Alzheimer's prognosis. With these findings, the physician prescribed two new medications for discharge:

Memantine (Namenda)—used to treat dementia associated with Alzheimer's disease

Donepezil (Aricept)—used for the treatment of mild to moderate Alzheimer's symptoms

Follow-up

☑ Self-Query: Possible Answers

In answer to the son and daughter's questions:

There is some evidence that vitamin E may slow the progression of Alzheimer's.

Studies are inconclusive about whether taking NSAIDs helps to slow the progression of Alzheimer's.

Studies are inconclusive about whether ginkgo biloba shows any results.

Case Study Inquiry

22

Vocabulary

🔎 Self-Query

Before attempting to work the case study, define each of the vocabulary words. Although the words may have several subheadings, it will give you a place to begin your inquiry.

Demyelination of the brain

_____

Diplopia

_____

Dysarthria

_____

Intention tremor

_____

Nystagmus

_____

Paresthesia

_____

Recent History

You are the nurse working for a neurologist who has ordered the biological response modifier interferon beta-1a (Avonex) for a patient. The patient has an appointment today to be taught about this new medication. Before the patient, a 26-year-old female, arrives in the office, you are reviewing her chart.

🔎 Self-Query

What do I know about the patient, given that she has been prescribed interferon beta-1a?

_____

_____

What is another name for interferon beta-1a? How is it administered? What are the uses for the medication? Are there any off-label uses?

_____

_____

Just before she is due to arrive at the office, you receive a call from her husband. He states that he has taken her to the emergency department. She is having problems with her eyesight and speech. He fears that she may be having a stroke. At the hospital, the patient undergoes a cerebral spinal fluid electrophoresis that reveals an increase in white blood cells, an increase in myelin basic protein, and the presence of IgG bands. The MRI reveals the presence of plaques.

Physician Orders I

Begin interferon beta-1a 30 mcg IM now and weekly (teaching for home)

Methylprednisolone (Solu-Medrol) 1 g IV daily for 3 days; consult a home infusion pharmacy for the possibility of home infusion

Amitriptyline (Elavil) 100 mg orally every 6 hours

Clonazepam (Klonopin) 1 mg orally at bedtime

Self-Query

Before consulting a pharmacology text, what do I know about these medications? What lab work needs to assessed with these medications?

Interferon beta-1a

_____

_____

Methylprednisolone

_____

_____

Amitriptyline

_____

_____

Clonazepam

_____

_____

Nursing Process

Self-Query

What nursing assessment should be performed regarding each medication? What planning and implementation do I need to do regarding each medication? How do I evaluate each medication's effectiveness?

Interferon beta-1a

_____

_____

Methylprednisolone

_____

_____

Amitriptyline

_____

_____

Clonazepam

_____

_____

Physician Orders II

The patient has had a partial recovery and will be sent home on the following medications:

Interferon beta-1a 30 mcg IM weekly

Amitriptyline 100 mg orally every 6 hours

Clonazepam 1 mg orally at bedtime

Methotrexate 2.5 mg every 12 hours × 3 doses over 36 hours every Wednesday at 6 a.m.

Increase baclofen 5 mg orally every 8 hours to 10 mg every 8 hours

Oxybutynin (Ditropan) 5 mg orally every 12 hours

Ibuprofen (Motrin) 800 mg every 12 hours as needed for pain

Self-Query

Before consulting a pharmacology text, what can you explain regarding these medications? Compare what you think you know with what is in the text. Do you know how these medications work? What lab work needs to be assessed regarding these medications?

Interferon beta-1a

_____

_____

Amitriptyline

_____

_____

Clonazepam

_____

_____

Methotrexate

_____

_____

Baclofen

_____

_____

Oxybutynin

_____

_____

Ibuprofen

_____

_____

Nursing Process

Self-Query

What nursing assessment should be performed for each medication? What planning and implementation do I need to do regarding each medication? How do I evaluate each medication's effectiveness?

Interferon beta-1a

_____

_____

Amitriptyline

_____

_____

Clonazepam

_____

_____

Methotrexate

_____

_____

Baclofen

_____

_____

Oxybutynin

_____

_____

Ibuprofen

_____

_____

Physician Orders III

Before leaving the hospital, the patient states that ibuprofen has given her an ulcer in the past, and she wants a drug ordered to keep her from developing another ulcer. The physician prescribes misoprostol (Cytotec) 100 mcg orally every 6 hours with meals. The physician also orders a pregnancy test.

Self-Query

Why did the physician order the pregnancy test? Which medications are contraindicated in pregnancy? Is misoprostol contraindicated in pregnancy?

_____

_____

Which pregnancy risk classification is misoprostol? What is the pharmacological class of misoprostol? What is misoprostol's therapeutic class?

_____

_____

Develop a teaching plan for the patient and her husband regarding her home medications.

_____

_____

_____

Develop two nursing diagnoses for this patient (NANDA).

_____

_____

Develop at least three patient outcomes (NOC).

_____

_____

Develop at least three patient interventions (NIC).

_____

_____

Synopsis

22

Because you can find answers to the self-queries in numerous texts, you will not find the answers to all of them here. However, you will find discussion of the individual case. The scenario relates to a 26-year-old female newly diagnosed with multiple sclerosis (MS); therefore, purposefully look into the medication use and vocabulary as they relate to these factors.

Vocabulary

When reviewing the vocabulary words, you might want to ask several questions: who, what, where, when, why, and how. This should give you a much broader understanding of each word.

Do yourself a favor and do not just give the shortest and simplest answer. Use the following example of demyelination of the brain: Instead of answering, "Demyelination of the brain is the loss of the myelin sheath insulating the nerves," ask:

What is the myelin sheath? Where is it located? Which medications alter the sheath? What is **demyelination of the brain**? Which medications are used in the treatment of demyelination? Which diseases are known for demyelination? What are the symptoms related to demyelination? How do anti-inflammatory medications appear to slow the progression of demyelination?

☑ Self-Query: Possible Answers

When defining the remainder of the vocabulary words, ask the following questions:

What is **diplopia**? How does this develop in MS patients? Who else is at risk of developing diplopia? Why does it develop?

What is **dysarthria**? How does dysarthria develop in MS patients? Who else is at risk of developing dysarthria? Why does it develop?

What is an **intention tremor**? How does it develop in MS patients? Who else is at risk of developing intention tremors?

What is **nystagmus**? How does nystagmus develop in MS patients? Who else is at risk of developing nystagmus? Why does it develop?

What is **paresthesia**? How does paresthesia develop in MS patients? Who else is at risk of developing paresthesia? Why does it develop?

Physician Orders I

☑ Self-Query: Possible Answers

Interferon beta-1a (Avonex) is prescribed to patients with relapsing forms of MS. It is hoped that the medication will decrease physical symptoms. The recommended dose is 30 mcg. The assessment exam and labs at the hospital reveal what the physician already knows; these results are expected in MS patients. The drug's exact mechanism of action is not known; however, it is known that interferon classifications work by decreasing the unwanted immune reaction against myelin.

Methylprednisolone (Solu-Medrol) is a liquid corticosteroid. It is prescribed for MS in high IV doses (100 mg daily for 3 days). It works by reducing the inflammation around a lesion and closing the blood–brain barrier. Note that the patient was taken to the hospital by her husband because of problems with her eyesight and speech. The methylprednisolone was infused as soon as the IV could be inserted. She was admitted for a 23-hour observation in the hospital on the neurological floor. The methylprednisolone was credited for clearing up her vision within 6 hours of the first treatment. The vision problems were diagnosed as optic neuritis.

Amitriptyline (Elavil) is a tricyclic antidepressant; this is a case of off-label use. It is used in MS patients to treat painful paresthesia (which is caused by damage in the brain and spinal cord) in the arms and legs.

Clonazepam (Klonopin) is a benzodiazepine used as a central nervous system (CNS) depressant, which slows down the nervous system. Clonazepam has numerous uses. It is used in MS patients primarily for the treatment of tremor, pain, and spasticity. It also decreases the anxiety that results from the disease process.

Physician Orders II

☑ Self-Query: Possible Answers

A GABA derivative, baclofen is a medication known to relax skeletal muscles. It is prescribed in MS patients to reduce spasticity. The patient was released after 23 hours, and a home infusion company was contacted to complete the next two doses of methylprednisolone.

Additional medications for home:

Oral methotrexate is a powerful immunosuppressant that has beneficial effects on relapse rates and delays disease progression in MS patients. Remember that it is also used in cancer therapy and should be treated as such.

Oxybutynin (Ditropan) is an antispasmodic. Remember that MS patients will have problems with muscle control during exacerbations of the disease. Bladder control is just one issue. The medication helps decrease muscle spasms of the bladder and the strong urge to urinate caused by these spasms.

Most individuals are familiar with ibuprofen (Motrin), an over-the-counter medication. It is a nonsteroidal anti-inflammatory (NSAID). It is used to relieve pain and reduce fever. One of its mechanisms of action appears to be the inhibition of prostaglandin production. Prostaglandins, as we know, are involved in the inflammatory process. In this case, there are two reasons for this medication: It is used to manage flulike symptoms caused by the interferon beta-1a, and for pain relief related to spasticity.

Physician Orders III

☑ Self-Query: Possible Answers

The physician ordered a pregnancy test because this drug causes uterine contractions that could lead to a miscarriage. This patient is of childbearing age and should be counseled on this medication.

Misoprostol (Cytotec) is pregnancy risk category X (can cause a miscarriage). The pharmacological class of misoprostol is prostaglandin E1 analogue. It protects gastric mucosa. Remember that prostaglandins help protect the stomach mucosa. NSAIDs decrease the production of prostaglandins.

Case Study Inquiry

23

Vocabulary

⁇ Self-Query

Before attempting to work the case study, define each of the vocabulary words. Although the words may have several subheadings, it will give you a place to begin your inquiry.

Enteral

_____

Exacerbation

_____

Hypoxemia

_____

Hypoxia

_____

Parenteral

_____

Percutaneous

_____

Pseudomonas

_____

Steroids

_____

A 75-year-old male is admitted to the emergency department in apparent respiratory distress.

Recent History

Two days ago, he was seen by his primary care provider and reported chills, a cough, and dyspnea with exertion. The physician prescribed:

Fluticasone and salmeterol inhaler (Advair Diskus)
Cefuroxime (Ceftin) 250 mg

⁇ Self-Query

Why did the physician order these two medications? How do they work?

Fluticasone and salmeterol inhaler

_____

_____

Cefuroxime

_____

_____

Unfortunately, the patient did not think he could afford the new medications and relied on the "stash" he saved at home. He used an old albuterol inhaler that he had saved and a leftover dose of Ceclor that was in his medicine cabinet. Write a teaching plan on why this is a bad idea. Give an explanation related to bacteria and the effects of time on the medication.

_____

_____

_____

The man returns today with worsening symptoms. You are now reviewing home medications with his wife and daughter.

Home Medications

Albuterol and ipratropium (Combivent) inhaled 18 mcg 2–3 puffs daily

Albuterol inhaler (in cabinet, expired 2 years ago)

Aspirin (ASA) 81 mg orally with lunch

Atorvastatin (Lipitor) 20 mg orally daily

Calcium carbonate (Tums) OTC 2 tabs chewed daily

Cefaclor (Ceclor) 500 mg (in cabinet, also expired 2 years ago)

Cefuroxime (Ceftin) 250 mg (he has the prescription but never filled it)

Celecoxib (Celebrex) 200 mg orally daily

Clopidogrel (Plavix) 75 mg orally daily

Docusate sodium OTC 100 mg 1 capsule orally daily as needed

Fluticasone and salmeterol inhaler (Advair Diskus) 250/50 (he has the prescription but never filled it)

Glipizide 10 mg orally daily

Guaifenesin 200 mg every 12 hours

Iron 27 mg orally daily

Metformin 500 mg orally twice daily

Pantoprazole 40 mg orally daily

Self-Query

Reviewing the medications, what are the patient's possible past medical diagnoses?

_____

_____

Do I know how these medications work? What lab work needs to be assessed with these medications?

Albuterol and ipratropium

_____

_____

Albuterol inhaler

_____

_____

Aspirin

_____

_____

Atorvastatin

_____

_____

Calcium carbonate

_____

_____

Cefaclor

_____

_____

Cefuroxime

_____

_____

Celecoxib

_____

_____

Clopidogrel

_____

_____

Docusate sodium

_____

_____

Fluticasone and salmeterol inhaler

_____

_____

Glipizide

_____

_____

Guaifenesin

_____

_____

Iron

_____

_____

Metformin

_____

_____

Pantoprazole

_____

_____

Nursing Process

Self-Query

What nursing assessment should I perform regarding each medication? What planning and implementation do I need to do for each medication? How do I evaluate each medication's effectiveness?

Albuterol and ipratropium

_____

_____

Albuterol inhaler

_____

_____

Aspirin

_____

_____

Atorvastatin

_____

_____

Calcium carbonate

_____

_____

Cefaclor

_____

_____

Cefuroxime

_____

_____

Celecoxib

_____

_____

Clopidogrel

_____

_____

Docusate sodium

_____

_____

Fluticasone and salmeterol inhaler

_____

_____

Glipizide

_____

_____

Guaifenesin

_____

_____

Iron

_____

_____

Metformin

_____

_____

Pantoprazole

_____

_____

Body Systems

Self-Query

Be prepared to defend your answers.

Can I place each medication under the body system that it commonly affects?

Neurological

_____

Cardiovascular

_____

Hematological

_____

Pulmonary

_____

Gastrointestinal

_____

Nutrition

_____

Genitourinary/renal

_____

Musculoskeletal
_____

Endocrine
_____

Integumentary
_____

Immune
_____

Pain/comfort
_____

The patient becomes unconscious. He develops bradycardia with a heart rate of 50, and his blood pressure is 80/40. You also see the beginning of rare premature ventricular beats on the screen.

Physical Assessment Findings
Neurological Assessment

Alert; oriented speech; clear grips, weak bilaterally; gait uneven

Cardiovascular and Hematological Assessment

BNP negative, K+ 3.9, S_1S_2 monitor reveals atrial fibrillation rate of 110

Blood pressure 156/90, generalized edema, capillary refill at 3 seconds

Slight click noted at aortic placement (later noted previous valve replacement 10 years prior)

RBC 2.70, Hgb 8.9, Hct 29.0, sodium 128, potassium 3.5, WBC 12.0

Pulmonary Assessment

Course inspiratory and expiratory rhonchi

Respiratory arrested in ER and now on ventilator PEEP of 12

Respiratory rate of 12, no spontaneous respirations

Green secretions noted in vent tubing

Chest x-ray revealed pneumonia

Sputum specimen revealed *Pseudomonas*

Gastrointestinal Assessment

Active bowel sounds, NGT inserted to low intermittent suction

Genitourinary Assessment

Foley, clear dark urine to bedside drainage bag at 50 mL/hr

Musculoskeletal Assessment

Sedated at present and not moving

Noted joint enlargement of hands

Endocrine Assessment

History of type II DM

Glucose 80

Integumentary Assessment

Warm, dry, pale

PICC line, right brachial area

Noted red areas to heels and toes

Immune Assessment

Compromised because of age

Pain/Comfort Assessment

Sedated and presently nonresponsive

Physician Orders I

Ipratropium (Atrovent) 0.02% nebulizer aerosol treatment every 6 hours

Esomeprazole (Nexium) 40 mg IV daily

One ampule MVI to 1000 mL NS daily at 125mL/hr

Lacri-Lube, one drop to each eye every 8 hours

Enoxaparin (Lovenox) 30 mg subcutaneously daily

Nystatin/triamcinolone (Mycolog) cream zinc oxide 1:1, apply to affected area

Regular insulin subcutaneously sliding scale

Methylprednisolone (Solu-Medrol) 125 mg IV every 6 hours

Fentanyl (Sublimaze) titrate as needed

   Supplied: fentanyl citrate 1000 mcg/20 mL in 100 mL of 5% dextrose

Propofol (Diprivan) titrate as needed

   Supplied: 1 g in 100 mL (10 mg/mL)

Ondansetron (Zofran) 4 mL IV every 4 hours as needed

Self-Query

Do I know how these medications work? What lab work needs to be assessed with these medications?

Ipratropium

_____

_____

Esomeprazole

_____

_____

One ampule MVI to 1000 mL NS

_____

_____

Lacri-Lube

_____

_____

Enoxaparin

_____

_____

Nystatin/triamcinolone

_____

_____

Regular insulin

_____

_____

Methylprednisolone

_____

_____

Fentanyl

_____

_____

Propofol

_____

_____

Ondansetron

_____

_____

Nursing Process

🜊 Self-Query

What nursing assessment should I perform for each medication? What planning and implementation do I need to do regarding each medication? How do I evaluate each medication's effectiveness?

Ipratropium

_____

_____

Esomeprazole

_____

_____

One ampule MVI to 1000 mL NS

_____

_____

Lacri-Lube

_____

_____

Enoxaparin

_____

_____

Nystatin/triamcinolone

_____

_____

Regular insulin

_____

_____

Methylprednisolone

_____

_____

Fentanyl

_____

_____

Propofol

_____

_____

Ondansetron

_____

_____

After 3 days, it is apparent that the patient will remain on the ventilator for a while longer. The NGT to LIS is replaced with a PEG tube.

Physician Orders II

Delivery through PEG tube

Pro-Stat 101 30 mg every 12 hours

Pulmocare

   First day: half strength, first 8 hours, 25 mL/hr; second 8 hours, 50 mL; third 8 hours, 75 mL/hr

   Second day: full strength at 75 mL/hr

Furosemide (Lasix) 40 mg NGT

Potassium 20 mEq 3 times a day

Captopril (Capoten) 25 mg twice a day per NGT

Docusate 100 mg twice a day

Is there an advantage to placing a PEG tube?

_____

_____

Is Pulmocare considered TPN or enteral nutrition? (Explain your answer.)

_____

_____

How will the continuous tube feeding affect the medication administration?

_____

_____

Do I know how these PEG tube medications work? What lab work needs to be assessed with these medications?

Pro-Stat

_____

_____

Pulmocare

_____

_____

Furosemide

_____

_____

Potassium

_____

_____

Captopril

_____

_____

Docusate

_____

_____

Which medications will most likely be stopped if diarrhea occurs?

_____

_____

Nursing Process

☞ **Self-Query**

What nursing assessment should I perform for each medication? What planning and implementation do I need to do regarding each medication? How do I evaluate each medication's effectiveness?

Pro-Stat

_____

_____

Pulmocare

_____

_____

Furosemide

_____

_____

Potassium

_____

_____

Captopril

_____

_____

Docusate

_____

_____

Develop two nursing diagnoses for this patient (NANDA).

_____

_____

_____

Develop at least three patient outcomes (NOC).

_____

_____

_____

Develop at least three patient interventions (NIC).

_____

_____

_____

Synopsis

23

Because you can find answers to the self-queries in numerous texts, you will not find the answers to all of them here. However, you will find discussion of the individual cases. The scenario relates to a 75-year-old male with respiratory failure; therefore, purposefully look into the medication use and vocabulary as they relate to these factors.

Vocabulary

When reviewing the vocabulary words, you might want to ask several questions: who, what, where, when, why, and how. This should give you a much broader understanding of each word.

Do yourself a favor and do not just give the shortest and simplest answer. Use the following example of enteral: Instead of answering, "Enteral is any part of the gastrointestinal tract," ask:

What is the meaning of the word **enteral**? Where is it located? How are medications administered here?

☑ Self-Query: Possible Answers

When defining the remainder of the vocabulary words, ask the following questions:

What is an **exacerbation**? How does an exacerbation of lung disease occur?

What is **hypoxemia**? What systems are altered? Who is at risk of developing hypoxemia? How are medications beneficial?

What is **hypoxia**? What systems are altered? Who is at risk of developing hypoxia? What medications are beneficial?

What is the meaning of the word **parenteral**? Where is it located? How are medications administered here?

What is **percutaneous**? Which procedures are done in this fashion?

What is *Pseudomonas*? Where is it usually acquired?

What classification is a **steroid**? Why would steroids be administered in an individual with respiratory distress? How would steroids treat an exacerbation of lung disease (e.g., asthma, COPD)?

Recent History

☑ Self-Query: Possible Answers

Fluticasone and salmeterol inhaler (Advair Diskus) is a combination medication and serves two purposes. It contains fluticasone, a steroid, which prevents inflammation. It also contains salmeterol, a bronchodilator, which relaxes bronchioles and improves gas exchange in the lungs.

Cefuroxime (Ceftin) is a broad-spectrum cephalosporin antibiotic. It is effective against pneumonia in the respiratory tract.

A few things to keep in mind when teaching the patient about the effects of bacteria and time on medication: If stored properly, most medications are safe until their expiration date. Proper storage means storing them in a cool, dry, dark place. It is ideal to have the temperature between 50°F and 75°F. This individual lived in the South and kept his home air conditioned to 85°F with a fan. His kitchen, where he kept his medications, was usually very hot and humid. The medications that he had stashed not only were out of date but also most likely had deteriorated and were more harmful than beneficial. Thus, he returned with worsening symptoms.

Home Medications

☑ Self-Query: Possible Answers

Reviewing the medications, the patient's possible past medical diagnoses are:

Albuterol and ipratropium (Combivent) inhaled 18 mcg 2–3 puffs daily: asthma/COPD
Albuterol inhaler (in medicine cabinet; expired 2 years ago): asthma/COPD
Aspirin (ASA) 81 mg orally with lunch: cardiovascular
Atorvastatin (Lipitor) 20 mg orally daily: hyperlipidemia
Calcium carbonate (Tums) OTC 2 tabs chewed daily: gastric reflux
Cefaclor (Ceclor) 500 mg (in cabinet; expired 2 years ago): respiratory infection
Cefuroxime 250 mg (has the prescription but never filled it): respiratory infection
Celecoxib (Celebrex) 200 mg orally daily: osteoarthritis
Clopidogrel (Plavix) 75 mg orally daily: cardiovascular
Docusate sodium OTC 100 mg 1 capsule orally daily as needed: constipation
Fluticasone and salmeterol inhaler 250/50 (has the prescription but never filled it): asthma/COPD
Glipizide 10 mg orally daily: type II diabetes
Guaifenesin 200 mg every 12 hours: respiratory/expectorant
Iron 27 mg orally daily: anemia
Metformin 500 mg orally twice daily: type II diabetes
Pantoprazole 40 mg orally daily: gastric reflux

See medication text for more details on how these medications work.

Body Systems

☑ Self-Query: Possible Answers

Neurological

None; however, keep in mind the diabetic medication and the fact that any medication can cause a neurological change.

Cardiovascular

Clopidogrel 75 mg orally daily
Atorvastatin 20 mg orally daily
Aspirin 81 mg orally with lunch

Hematological

Clopidogrel 75 mg orally daily
Atorvastatin 20 mg orally daily
Aspirin 81 mg orally with lunch
Iron 27 mg orally daily

OTC calcium carbonate 2 tabs chewed daily (He takes calcium carbonate for GI issues but should realize that it is calcium, which can alter hematological and cardiac functions.)

Pulmonary

Fluticasone and salmeterol 250/50 (has the prescription but never filled it)
Albuterol and ipratropium inhaled 18 mcg 2–3 puffs daily
Albuterol inhaler (in cabinet; expired 2 years ago)
Guaifenesin 200 mg every 12 hours
Placed in the system of infection:
   Cefuroxime 250 mg
   Cefaclor 500 mg (in cabinet; expired 2 years ago)

Gastrointestinal

Pantoprazole 40 mg orally daily
OTC calcium carbonate 2 tabs chewed daily
OTC docusate sodium 100 mg 1 capsule orally daily as needed
Iron 27 mg orally daily: Although it is taken for anemia, individuals need to be aware that one of its main side effects is constipation.

Nutrition

Iron 27 mg orally daily

Genitourinary/renal

None

Musculoskeletal

Celecoxib 200 mg orally daily
Osteoarthritis

Endocrine

Some of you may place the diabetic medications here. Look to see what the mechanism of action actually is. Do they alter the pancreas? Do they alter cellular function in regard to glucose?
Glipizide 10 mg orally daily
Metformin 500 mg orally twice daily

Integumentary

None

Immune

None

Pain/comfort

Although there are no actual pain relief medications in the patient's sack, he probably does take an occasional OTC pain reliever. Also be aware that all these medications are used to decrease the discomfort of his disease process.

Physician Orders I

☑ Self-Query: Possible Answers

Ipratropium (Atrovent) is used for the symptomatic management of bronchospasms associated with COPD. Note that the inhaler the patient attempted to use expired 2 years ago. He also had several other pulmonary medications. This patient has a long history of pulmonary disease.

Esomeprazole (Nexium) and other proton pump inhibitors are a mainstay for acute acid suppression in hospitalized patients. Stress ulceration generally begins in the proximal regions of the stomach within hours of major trauma or serious illness.

Nutritional support: Further investigation revealed the following ingredients in the MVI bag: vitamins A and D, riboflavin (B2), ascorbic acid (C), thiamine (B1), pyridoxine (B6), niacin, vitamin B5, vitamin E, biotin (B7), folic acid (B9), and folate (vitamin B12). He received it for nutritional deficiency and *Pseudomonas* pneumonia, and because of his age. No vitamin deficiencies were clinically evident; however, this situation placed severe stress on his body's metabolic demands and depleted his body of nutrients. Further investigation revealed the ingredients. Many hospitals refer to the MVI bag as a banana bag because of its yellow color.

Lacri-Lube helps to prevent corneal abrasion in paralyzed and ventilated/sedated individuals.

Enoxaparin (Lovenox) is a prophylaxis treatment for the prevention of deep vein thrombosis.

Nystatin/triamcinolone (Mycolog): After the intubation, the nurse reported a red, inflamed groin area covering the testicles and base of the penis. IV Diflucan may also be an intervention if the patient does not respond.

Regular insulin: Note that the medications are usually placed in dextrose. Ask the pharmacist if they are compatible with normal saline, and have them placed in that fluid for infusion; this will help to keep the glucose levels within range. There must be tight glucose control; evidence has shown that effective glucose control in the intensive care unit decreases morbidity across a broad range of conditions and decreases mortality. Check to see if these IV medications are compatible.

Methylprednisolone (Solu-Medrol) is a corticosteroid that will alter the inflammatory response used here for the lungs; glucose levels and the growth of the *Candida* will need to be monitored.

Supplied: Fentanyl citrate 1000 mcg/20 mL in 100 mL of 5% dextrose. Fentanyl (Sublimaze) is considered a short-acting narcotic analgesic and is the preferred analgesic agent for critically ill patients with hemodynamic instability. It causes respiratory depression in this form, so the patient must be on a ventilator.

Supplied: 1 gram in 100 mL (10 mg/mL). Propofol (Diprivan) is a short-acting sedative-hypnotic IV agent. It is used for inducing general anesthesia, in the maintenance of general anesthesia, and in sedation for intubated, mechanically ventilated adults in critical care units. Propofol is not considered an analgesic, so you will see it used in this case with fentanyl for pain control. Watch for hepatic side effects; the mixture of the actual drug propofol, soybean oil, and purified egg lecithin is a great medium for bacteria. It also has an additive that inhibits microbial growth.

Ondansetron (Zofran) is an antiemetic that works by blocking serotonin receptors in the chemoreceptor trigger zone (CTZ). After 3 days, it is apparent that the patient will remain on the ventilator for a while longer. The NGT to LIS is replaced with a PEG tube.

Physician Orders II

☑ Self-Query: Possible Answers

Delivery through PEG tube.

The order for Pro-Stat had to be clarified because it is a liquid and is delivered in liquid form (30 mL, not mg). Speaking to the pharmacist revealed why it was ordered: This 30 mL (1 oz) has 15 grams of protein. The protein helps promote tissue healing and weight stabilization. It is used for PEG tubes because it does not clog them. Remember that this individual has pneumonia and COPD, so his requirements for protein and other nutrition such as calories are increased.

Pulmocare: First day: 1/2 strength, first 8 hours, 25 mL/hr; second 8 hours, 50 mL; third 8 hours, 75 mL/hr. Second day: full strength at 75 mL/hr. After consulting with the dietician, you discover the reason for enteral feeding (as opposed to other methods): It has high calories and decreased carbohydrates. The decreased carbohydrates decreased the production of CO_2, which is very helpful in individuals with COPD.

Furosemide (Lasix) is a diuretic to promote fluid homeostasis.

Monitor potassium levels with furosemide.

Captopril (Capoten) was ordered because the individual became hypertensive. He was also monitored through a pulmonary artery catheter. The physician believed that administration of an ACE inhibitor would lower blood pressure and improve his pulmonary function.

Docusate is used to treat or prevent constipation. It helps to draw fluids into the intestine to mix with the stool. Monitor for loose stools.

There is an advantage to placing a PEG tube. This individual will need added nutrition while on the ventilator, and having a nasogastric tube will be very irritating to the skin.

This man survived.

Case Study Inquiry

24

Vocabulary

Self-Query

Before attempting to work the case study, define each of the vocabulary words. Although the words may have several subheadings, it will give you a place to begin your inquiry.

Atrial flutter

_____

Buccal

_____

Cardiac tamponade

_____

Intermittent claudication

_____

Nocturia

_____

Orthostatic hypotension

_____

Oxygen saturation

_____

Petechiae

_____

Pulsus paradoxus

_____

Splinter hemorrhage

_____

A 58-year-old male is admitted to the emergency department with chest pain that is radiating down his right arm. Twenty-four hours earlier, he was seen in the same emergency room for severe indigestion and belching. He has a history of gastroesophageal reflux disease (GERD). An ECG was performed without revealing any changes.

Physician Orders I

Physician prescribes a mixture consisting of:

Aluminum/magnesium (Maalox) 30 mL

Belladonna alkaloids/phenobarbital (Donnatal) 5 mL

Xylocaine (Lidocaine Viscous) 20 mL

Why were these medications ordered? Do I know how these medications work? What lab work needs to be assessed with these medications?

Aluminum/magnesium

_____

_____

Belladonna alkaloids/phenobarbital

_____

_____

Xylocaine

_____

_____

Is there another name for this combination?

_____

_____

Nursing Process

🜂 **Self-Query**

What nursing assessment should I perform regarding each medication? What planning and implementation do I need to do regarding each medication? How do I evaluate each medication's effectiveness?

Aluminum/magnesium

_____

_____

Belladonna alkaloids/phenobarbital

_____

_____

Xylocaine

_____

_____

Follow-up

After 1 hour, his pain was relieved and he went home. This morning, he awoke with chest pain and pain radiating down his left arm. He is also diaphoretic and nauseated. You are now in a code situation as the man becomes unconscious and is placed on a ventilator. He now has ST segment elevations on the EKG. You remember the man from the previous day and call for the previous day's chart, along with any old charts. It is then that you realize he was not totally honest the previous day when he said that his only medical history was GERD.

Home Medications

Noted on old chart:

Aspirin (ASA) 325 mg every morning

Famotidine (Pepcid) 20 mg orally daily

Furosemide (Lasix) 40 mg orally daily

Hydrocodone bitartrate and acetaminophen (Lorcet) 10 mg every 8 hours as needed

Ipratropium (Atrovent) 2 puffs inhaled at 9 a.m. and 9 p.m. (every 12 hours)

Methocarbamol (Robaxin) 750 orally 3 times a day

Nitroglycerin (Nitro-Dur) 6.5 mg orally every 8 hours

Pregabalin (Lyrica) 50 mg orally twice a day

Ramipril 5 mg orally daily

Repaglinide (Prandin) 1 mg twice a day

Sertraline (Zoloft) 150 mg orally daily

Slo-Bid 300 mg orally 3 times a day

☞ Self-Query

Using a drug book or pharmacology text that contains the mechanism of action, unlabeled uses, and pharmacokinetics for medications, answer the following questions. Make answers specific to this scenario.

What do I know about these medications? For each medication, what is the recommended dose, recommended route, and best time of day to give it? Do I know what lab results I need in regard to each medication? Do I know the approved use of each medication? Do I know the most common diseases treated by the listed medications? Are any off-label uses approved for each drug?

Aspirin

_____

_____

Famotidine

_____

_____

Furosemide

_____

_____

Hydrocodone bitartrate and acetaminophen

_____

_____

Ipratropium

_____

_____

Methocarbamol

_____

_____

Nitroglycerin

_____

_____

Pregabalin

_____

_____

Ramipril

_____

_____

Repaglinide

_____

_____

Sertraline

_____

_____

Slo-Bid

_____

_____

Do I know the individual's past medical history by looking at the medication list?

_____

_____

Body Systems

Self-Query

Be prepared to defend your answers.

Can I place each medication under the body system that it commonly affects?

Neurological

_____

Cardiovascular

_____

Hematological

_____

Pulmonary

_____

Gastrointestinal

_____

Nutrition

_____

Genitourinary/renal

_____

Musculoskeletal

_____

Endocrine

_____

Integumentary

_____

Immune

_____

Pain/comfort

_____

Thinking back to the previous day, if the patient was having angina at the time, why did the "GI cocktail" relieve the gastric pain?

_____

_____

Nursing Process

Self-Query

Do I know how these medications work? What nursing assessment will I perform regarding each medication? What planning and implementation do I need to do for each medication? How do I evaluate each medication's effectiveness?

Aspirin

_____

_____

Famotidine

_____

_____

Furosemide

_____

_____

Hydrocodone bitartrate and acetaminophen

_____

_____

Ipratropium

_____

_____

Methocarbamol

_____

_____

Nitroglycerin

_____

_____

Pregabalin

_____

_____

Ramipril

_____

_____

Repaglinide

_____

_____

Sertraline

_____

_____

Slo-Bid

_____

_____

Physical Assessment Findings
Neurological Assessment

Sedated while on ventilator, pupils reactive to light

Cardiovascular and Hematological Assessment

Troponin 1, 2.2; BNP 900 picograms/mL, K+ 4.9; $S_1S_2S_3$
Monitor reveals atrial flutter with 4:1 conduction
Blood pressure 90/50, trace lower extremity edema, capillary refill at 3 seconds
Hgb, 15, Hct, 48.0, sodium 135

Pulmonary Assessment

Course rhonchi throughout
Ventilator PEEP of 5 (saturation of 96%)
Respiratory rate of 14

Gastrointestinal Assessment

Active bowel sounds, weight 280 pounds, height 5'8"

Genitourinary Assessment

Foley clear urine to bedside drainage bag at 30 mL/hr
Creatinine 2.9

Musculoskeletal Assessment

Large muscular arms; wife states history of back injury from lifting hay on their farm

Endocrine Assessment

History of type II DM

Glucose 170

Integumentary Assessment

Warm, dry, pale PA line inserted to right chest area

Arterial line to left radial artery

No bruising noted

Immune Assessment

Wife denies that her husband had difficulty fighting off colds or viruses

Pain/Comfort Assessment

Sedated and presently nonresponsive

Physician Orders II

Ipratropium (Atrovent) 0.02% nebulizer aerosol treatment every 6 hours

Esomeprazole (Nexium) 40 mg IV daily

Lacri-Lube one drop to each eye every 8 hours

Regular insulin subcutaneously sliding scale

Heparin to arterial line

Heparin 25,000 units/250 mL NS at 18 mL/hr

Norepinephrine to keep MAP 60–70

Fentanyl (Sublimaze) titrate as needed

   Supplied: fentanyl citrate 1000 mcg/20 mL in 100 mL of 5% dextrose

Propofol (Diprivan) titrate as needed

   Supplied: 1 gram in 100 mL (10 mg/mL)

Ondansetron (Zofran) IV 4 mL every 4 hours as needed

Morphine sulfate 2–4 mg pain

Mix 50 mg nitroglycerin in 250 mL D_5W

   Start: 10–20 mcg/min (3–6 mL/hour)

Self-Query

Do I know how these medications work? What lab work needs to be assessed with these medications?

Ipratropium

_____

_____

Esomeprazole

_____

_____

Lacri-Lube

_____

_____

Regular insulin

_____

_____

Heparin

_____

_____

Norepinephrine

_____

_____

Fentanyl

_____

_____

Propofol

_____

_____

Ondansetron

_____

_____

Morphine sulfate

_____

_____

Nitroglycerin

_____

_____

_____

Nursing Process

? Self-Query

What nursing assessment should I perform for each medication? What planning and implementation do I need to do regarding each medication? How do I evaluate each medication's effectiveness?

Ipratropium

_____

_____

Esomeprazole

_____

_____

Lacri-Lube

_____

_____

Regular insulin

_____

_____

Heparin

_____

_____

Norepinephrine

_____

_____

Fentanyl

_____

_____

Propofol

_____

_____

Ondansetron

_____

_____

Morphine sulfate

_____

_____

Nitroglycerin

_____

_____

Develop two nursing diagnoses for this patient (NANDA).

_____

_____

Develop at least three patient outcomes (NOC).

_____

_____

_____

Develop at least three patient interventions (NIC).

_____

_____

_____

Develop two nursing diagnoses for this family (NANDA).

_____

_____

Develop at least three family outcomes (NOC).

_____

_____

_____

Develop at least three family interventions (NIC).

_____

_____

_____

Synopsis

24

Because you can find answers to the self-queries in numerous texts, you will not find the answers to all of them here. However, you will find discussion of the individual case. The scenario relates to cardiogenic shock in critical care; therefore, purposefully look into the medication use and vocabulary as they relate to these factors.

Vocabulary

When reviewing the vocabulary words, you might want to ask several questions: who, what, where, when, why, and how. This should give you a much broader understanding of each word.

Do yourself a favor and do not just give the shortest and simplest answer. Use the following example of buccal: Instead of answering, "Buccal is a way to administer medications orally," ask:

What is **buccal**? Who can use this route? Which medications can be delivered via this route?

☑ Self-Query: Possible Answers

When defining the remainder of the vocabulary words, ask the following questions:

Who is at risk for **atrial flutter**? What medications treat this? Why is it dangerous? What does it indicate?

How does **cardiac tamponade** develop? Who is at risk for this development? Which medications are used to treat it?

What is **intermittent claudication**? Who is at risk? How is it treated?

What is **nocturia**? Who is at risk? How is it treated?

What is **orthostatic hypotension**? Who is at risk? How is it treated?

How is **oxygen saturation** measured?

What are **petechiae**? What medications cause it? Who is at risk? How is it treated?

What is **pulsus paradoxus**? What medications cause it? Who is at risk? How is it treated?

What are **splinter hemorrhages**? What medications cause it? Who is at risk? How is it treated?

Physician Orders I

☑ Self Query: Possible Answers

Aluminum/magnesium (Maalox) is an antacid used to reduce possible heartburn. Belladonna alkaloids/phenobarbital (Donnatal) is a combination medication, consisting of phenobarbital, hyoscyamine, atropine, and scopolamine. Xylocaine (Lidocaine Viscous) is a local anesthetic/pain relief agent.

This combination is also known as a GI cocktail.

The planning and implementation for each medication should be discussed with an instructor and in a group.

When assessing the effectiveness of a medication, see the reason the medication was prescribed.

Home Medications

Aspirin (ASA) 325 mg every morning: platelets

Famotidine (Pepcid) 20 mg orally daily: heartburn

Furosemide (Lasix) 40 mg orally daily: fluid

Hydrocodone bitartrate and acetaminophen (Lorcet) 10 mg every 8 hours as needed: analgesic

Ipratropium (Atrovent) 2 puffs inhaled at 9 a.m. and 9 p.m. (every 12 hours): bronchospasm prevention (not treatment)

Methocarbamol (Robaxin) 750 mg orally 3 times a day: muscle relaxer

Nitroglycerin (Nitro-Dur) 6.5 mg orally every 8 hours: chest pain

Pregabalin (Lyrica) 50 mg orally twice a day: analgesic

Ramipril 5 mg orally daily: hypertension

Repaglinide (Prandin) 1 mg two times a day: lowers glucose levels, used in type II diabetes

Sertraline (Zoloft) 150 mg orally daily: depression

Slo-Bid 300 mg orally 3 times a day: shortness of breath

Discuss the patient's possible past medical diagnoses and the lab work that needs to be assessed in groups, being sure to note the patient's physical findings.

Body Systems

☑ **Self-Query: Possible Answers**

Neurological

Sertraline 150 mg orally daily (SSRI)
Pregabalin 50 mg orally twice a day
Hydrocodone bitartrate and acetaminophen 10 mg every 8 hours as needed
Methocarbamol 750 orally three times a day

Cardiovascular

Nitroglycerin 6.5 mg orally every 8 hours
Aspirin 325 mg every morning
Ramipril 5 mg orally daily
Furosemide 40 mg orally daily
See Donnatal ingredients; would any have a cardiac effect?

Hematological

Aspirin

Pulmonary

Ipratropium 2 puffs inhaled at 9 a.m. and 9 p.m. (every 12 hours)
Slo-Bid 300 mg orally 3 times a day (will affect cardiac status)

Gastrointestinal

Famotidine 20 mg orally daily

Nutrition

Repaglinide 1 mg twice a day

Genitourinary/renal

Ramipril 5 mg orally daily
Furosemide 40 mg orally daily

Musculoskeletal

Methocarbamol 750 orally 3 times a day

Endocrine

Some might place repaglinide here. Look to see if it actually works on the pancreas or modifies cellular structure for the uptake of glucose.

Integumentary

None specific

Immune

None specific

Pain/comfort

Methocarbamol 750 orally 3 times a day
Pregabalin 50 mg orally twice a day
Hydrocodone bitartrate and acetaminophen 10 mg every 8 hours as needed
Although these are specific for pain, the patient's medications (as all medications) are given to produce relief from the symptoms of the disease process.

Cardiac pain is sometimes relieved with a GI cocktail. Unfortunately, we may develop a false sense of security when the individual is experiencing a non–elevated ST segment myocardial infarction. It is more important to promote obtaining adequate history/background and examination skills. This would lead to the evaluation of cardiac risk factors and the findings of chest pain, and not, as in this individual's case, the diagnosis of GI distress.

Nursing Process

☑ Self-Query: Possible Answers

Review the mechanism of action and reason for giving to know how these medications work.

This patient did not have to progress to this stage. His heartburn was actually an untreated non-ST-elevated myocardial infarction (NSTEMI). He developed cardiac failure related to damaged heart muscle.

Physician Orders II

☑ Self Query: Possible Answers

Ipratropium is used for the symptomatic management of bronchospasms associated with COPD. In this individual, the problem was compounded because of his lung disease.

Proton pump inhibitors such as esomeprazole (Nexium) are a mainstay for acute acid suppression in hospitalized patients. Stress ulceration generally begins in the proximal regions of the stomach within hours of major trauma or serious illness.

Lacri-Lube helps to prevent corneal abrasion in paralyzed and ventilated/sedated individuals.

Regular insulin: Please note that the medications are usually placed in dextrose. Ask the pharmacist if the medications are compatible with normal saline, and have them placed in that fluid for infusion. Glucose control must be tight. Evidence has shown that effective glucose control in the ICU has been shown to decrease morbidity across a broad range of conditions and to decrease mortality.

Heparin: Anticoagulation keeps the line from clotting. This line is placed directly into the radial artery. It assists in blood pressure measurement and is used for withdrawing labs (arterial blood gases). The fewer puncture sites, the better, because the patient is also receiving heparin. Assess for compatibility of IV solutions and medications.

Heparin/normal saline: Anticoagulant—monitor vital signs, aPTT, Hgb, Hct, platelet count. Hemorrhage is always a possibility. Protamine should always be available.

Norepinephrine administration began during the cardiac arrest in the emergency department and has continued. Infusing through the large central line (pulmonary artery catheter) is a major catecholamine (others: epinephrine, dopamine, and dobutamine). It produces cardiovascular support to assist in the delivery of oxygen, thus the order to maintain the mean arterial pressure between 60 and 70; this keeps hemodynamic pressures at a level that allows for appropriate distribution of cardiac output for adequate tissue perfusion.

Fentanyl (Sublimaze) is considered a short-acting narcotic analgesic and is the preferred analgesic agent for critically ill patients with hemodynamic instability. It causes respiratory depression in this form, so the patient must be on a ventilator.

Propofol (Diprivan) is a short-acting sedative-hypnotic IV agent. It is used for inducing general anesthesia, in the maintenance of general anesthesia, and in sedation for intubated, mechanically ventilated adults in critical care units. Propofol is not considered an analgesic, so you will see it used in this case with fentanyl for pain control. Watch for hepatic side effects; the mixture of the actual drug propofol, soybean oil, and purified egg lecithin is a great medium for bacteria. It also has an additive that inhibits microbial growth.

Ondansetron (Zofran) is an antiemetic that works by blocking serotonin receptors in the chemoreceptor trigger zone (CTZ).

Although morphine sulfate is the opiate analgesic used for chest pain, it is always wise to begin the use of nitroglycerin for the chest pain. Morphine also assists in decreasing preload.

Nitroglycerin is a potent vasodilator. It allows oxygen-deprived tissue such as the heart and other organs to receive oxygen-rich blood. It decreases the heart's workload and oxygen demand.

NANDA/NIC/NOC can be discussed in a group setting guided by the instructor.

The patient did survive.

Case Study Inquiry

25

Vocabulary

Self-Query

Before attempting to work the case study, define each of the vocabulary words. Although the words may have several subheadings, it will give you a place to begin your inquiry.

Anticholinergics

_____

Arthroscopy

_____

Depression

_____

Gout

_____

Prostaglandins

_____

Steroids

_____

Stevens-Johnson syndrome

_____

Uric acid

_____

A 70-year-old male is admitted to the orthopedic floor with severe pain reported in his hands, feet, and right knee. He has a history of joint inflammation and has taken NSAIDs over the years to reduce the pain. However, this pain seems relentless; he presented to his primary care provider for care and is now admitted to your unit.

Home Medications

According to the patient's list:

Aspirin (Ecotrin) 325 mg every 8 hours as needed for pain

Calcium carbonate (Tums) ES 500 mg 2 tabs as needed for indigestion

Diphenhydramine 25 mg for sleep

Ibuprofen 200 mg every 8 hours as needed for pain

Omega-3 1000 mg 1 tab every morning with food

? Self-Query

Using a drug book or pharmacology text that contains the mechanism of action, unlabeled uses, and pharmacokinetics for medications, answer the following questions. Make answers specific to this scenario.

Are these prescription or over-the-counter medications?

_____

What qualifies the need to make a medication prescription only?

_____

What is the mechanism of action for these medications? What lab work needs to be assessed for this patient regarding the medications? What are the pharmacological classes of the listed medications? What are the therapeutic classes of the listed medications? How will I measure the effectiveness of each medication? How does the patient measure the effectiveness of the medications? Are the two measurements sometimes different?

Aspirin

_____

_____

_____

Calcium carbonate

_____

_____

_____

Diphenhydramine

_____

_____

_____

Ibuprofen

_____

_____

_____

Omega-3

_____

_____

_____

How do NSAIDs affect the kidneys?

_____

_____

How does a salicylate affect the kidneys?

_____

_____

How does aspirin affect prostaglandins? What effect does this have on the kidneys?

_____

_____

What are two medical uses for diphenhydramine?

_____

_____

What are two medical uses for omega-3 and calcium carbonate?

_____

_____

Is diphenhydramine the drug of choice for the geriatric patient to use for sleep?

_____

_____

Body Systems

Self-Query

Be prepared to defend your answers.

Can I place each medication under the body system that it commonly affects?

Neurological
_____

Cardiovascular
_____

Hematological
_____

Pulmonary
_____

Gastrointestinal
_____

Nutrition
_____

Genitourinary/renal
_____

Musculoskeletal
_____

Endocrine
_____

Integumentary
_____

Immune
_____

Pain/comfort
_____

Physical Assessment Findings
Neurological Assessment

Alert, talkative, pupils reactive to light

Grips moderately strong, reports pain with movement of hands and walking

Gait even, no signs of shuffle

Cardiovascular and Hematological Assessment

S_1S_2

Monitor reveals sinus at 78

Blood pressure 100/50, trace edema to lower extremities

Capillary refill at 3 seconds

Noted bruising to arms and legs (patient states that sometimes he bumps into things but does not fall)

Pulmonary Assessment

Lungs clear throughout

Respiratory rate of 18, respirations even and unlabored

Gastrointestinal Assessment

Active bowel sounds, weight 150 pounds, height 5'8"

Genitourinary Assessment

Patient states, "A little problem starting, but otherwise OK."

Obtaining 24-hour urinary uric acid

BUN 30, creatinine 1.1

Musculoskeletal Assessment

The patient states that he walks a mile every day and carries a 2-lb weight in each hand when he walks. However, for the past 5 days, has not been able to walk the mile or work with weights because of increasing pain.

Erythema and heat noted to finger joints

Tophi, subcutaneous nodules noted to hands and feet

ESR 28, serum uric acid 12/dL

Endocrine Assessment

Denies problem

Integumentary Assessment

Warm, dry, noted bruising as mentioned

IV normal saline at 50 to right forearm

Immune Assessment

Takes flu vaccine and has not had a cold in 5 years

Pain/Comfort Assessment

Noticeable grimace when asked to squeeze hands during assessment

Physician Orders

Stop all medications from home

Dietary consult

IV normal saline at 125 mL/hr

Colchicine 2 mg IV now and 0.5 mg IV in 6 hours
Reevaluate pain after 0.5 mg and call physician for further colchicine orders

On Day 2, begin:

Allopurinol 100 mg daily orally

Probenecid 250 mg daily

Acetaminophen/codeine #2 1–2 tabs orally every 4 hours for pain not relieved by colchicine

Self-Query

After assessing the physician's new orders, do I have an idea what the patient's diagnosis is?

_____

_____

Do I know how these medications work? What lab work needs to be assessed with these medications? What is the classification of each medication? Why is each medication usually given? How is it given? Do I know why the physician ordered each medication for this individual?

Colchicine

_____

_____

Allopurinol

_____

_____

Probenecid

_____

_____

Acetaminophen/codeine

_____

_____

Why reassess for pain after the second dose of colchicine?

_____

How much codeine is in this prescribed dose of medication?

_____

Nursing Process

What nursing assessment should I perform regarding each medication? What planning and implementation do I need to do regarding each medication? How do I evaluate each medication's effectiveness?

Colchicine

_____

_____

Allopurinol

_____

_____

Probenecid

_____

_____

Acetaminophen/codeine

_____

_____

Develop two nursing diagnoses for this patient (NANDA).

_____

_____

Develop at least three patient outcomes (NOC).

_____

_____

Develop at least three patient interventions (NIC).

_____

_____

Develop two nursing diagnoses for this family (NANDA).

_____

_____

Develop at least three family outcomes (NOC).

_____

_____

Develop at least three family interventions (NIC).

_____

_____

Dietary calls and asks for more information on the referral. Using the SBAR, what will I need to tell them?

_____

_____

_____

Synopsis

25

Because you can find answers to the self-queries in numerous texts, you will not find the answers to all of them here. However, you will find discussion of the individual case. The scenario relates to NSAIDs and gout; therefore, purposefully look into the medication use and vocabulary as they relate to these factors.

Vocabulary

When reviewing the vocabulary words, you might want to ask several questions: who, what, where, when, why, and how. This should give you a much broader understanding of each word.

Do yourself a favor and do not just give the shortest and simplest answer. Use the following example of prostaglandins: Instead of answering, "Prostaglandins are substances found in the lining of the stomach," ask:

Who discovered **prostaglandins**? Where are they located? What medications alter the function of prostaglandins?

☑ Self-Query: Possible Answers

When defining the remainder of the vocabulary words, ask the following questions:

What are **anticholinergics**? How do they work?

What is an **arthroscopy**? What can it tell us?

What is a cause of **depression**? How do steroids cause depression? How do medications treat depression?

What is **gout**? Who is at risk for gout? What medications promote the development of gout?

Who discovered **steroids**? Where are they produced in the body? How are steroids administered? What medications alter the function of steroids? What is a major side effect of steroid use? Why must they be tapered after long term use?

What is **Stevens-Johnson syndrome**? Who is at risk for this? What medications can cause this? How is it treated?

What is **uric acid**? How is it produced? What medications promote the development of uric acid? Which medications treat uric acid?

Home Medications

☑ Self-Query: Possible Answers

All these medications can be bought over the counter.

Ibuprofen is a nonsteroidal anti-inflammatory drug (NSAID). The patient uses ibuprofen for mild to moderate joint pain and inflammation, which are due to the release of prostaglandins. Ibuprofen blocks the enzyme that makes prostaglandins; this results in lower levels of prostaglandins, thus reducing pain and inflammation. The patient has used ibuprofen for 20 years.

Also known as enteric-coated aspirin, Ecotrin is an NSAID. The patient uses it for mild to moderate joint pain and inflammation, which are due to the release of prostaglandins. Aspirin blocks the enzyme that makes prostaglandins; this results in lower levels of prostaglandins, thus reducing pain and inflammation. Aspirin can also alter the blood uric acid level and should not be taken by anyone who has gout.

Calcium carbonate (Tums) is an antacid that neutralizes gastric acid and raises the pH in the stomach.

Diphenhydramine is an antihistamine and also blocks the action of acetylcholine. It can be used as a sedative because it causes drowsiness. It is not the drug of choice for geriatric individuals.

Omega-3 fatty acids are considered essential fatty acids. They are essential to human health but cannot be manufactured by the body. There are three major types of omega-3 fatty acids used by the body: ALA, EPA, and DHA.

Body Systems

☑ Self Query: Possible Answers

Neurological

  Diphenhydramine

Cardiovascular

  Omega-3 1000 mg

Hematological

  None specifically; however, note the alterations for omega-3 1000 mg.

Pulmonary

  None specifically

Gastrointestinal

  Calcium carbonate; note the effect of NSAIDs on the gastric lining in regard to prostaglandins.

Nutrition

  None specifically; however, note the alterations for omega-3 1000 mg.

Genitourinary/renal

  Note the effect that the use of NSAIDs has on the renal system.

Musculoskeletal

  The patient used his pain relievers mostly for this system.

Endocrine

  None specifically

Integumentary

  None specifically

Immune

  None specifically

Pain/comfort

  Ibuprofen 200 mg every 8 hours as needed for pain; aspirin 325 mg every 8 hours as needed for pain

Physician Orders

☑ Self-Query: Possible Answers

After reviewing the assessment and the patient's use of his medications at home, one can see a pattern of musculoskeletal issues.

To know how these medications work and what lab work needs to be assessed with the medications, the reader should look to lab results and the past diet of the patient.

Dietary consult: The individual needs counsel regarding an antigout diet.

IV normal saline at 125 mL/hr needed for hydration

Colchicine IV is used for the treatment of acute gout. It is an anti-inflammatory medication and was given via IV so the individual would not experience GI side effects, which are among its principal adverse effects. In addition, the IV route works faster.

The primary use of allopurinol is to treat excessive uric acid, which leads to the painful condition we know as gout. Allopurinol does not alleviate acute attacks of gout, but it is useful for chronic gout to help prevent future attacks. This is the reason for the dose following the colchicine. In addition, it can be used in individuals with kidney insufficiency.

Probenecid increases the excretion of uric acid in the kidneys so that it can be excreted in the urine. It is primarily used in treating gout. This medication is not to be given with aspirin because aspirin has been shown to decrease the effect of probenecid. Probenecid also blocks the excretion of some medications, elevating their levels in the blood. This altered excretion is seen with antibiotics (which can be beneficial by prolonging the effects) and with some NSAIDs (which can be very toxic and thus detrimental). This is the reason that the provider stopped all the home medications and placed the patient on Tylenol #2 (the medication listed next).

Acetaminophen is taken as a pain reliever, and codeine has similar properties to morphine and is prescribed for moderate to severe pain. The number next to the codeine indicates the amount of codeine added to the acetaminophen; it can range from 15 mg to 60 mg in the United States.

Just a reminder: NSAIDs are anti-inflammatories; acetaminophen is not. NSAIDS can damage the kidneys and cause gastrointestinal bleeding. Prolonged or chronic use of acetaminophen, which is metabolized in the liver, can result in liver failure.

Nursing Process

☑ Self Query: Possible Answers

Discuss NANDA, NIC, and NOC in groups.

Also discuss what you will tell dietary (using the SBAR) about the referral in groups.

The individual was sent home on:

> Allopurinol 100 mg daily orally
> Probenecid 250 mg daily orally
> Acetaminophen/codeine #2 1–2 tabs orally every 4–6 hours as needed for moderate to severe joint pain
> Omega-3 1000 mg 1 tab every morning with food

The patient was also instructed to use ibuprofen 200 mg every 8 hours as needed for mild pain and other pain not related to his joints.

Case Study Inquiry

26

Vocabulary

℗ Self-Query

Before attempting to work the case study, define each of the vocabulary words. Although the words may have several subheadings, it will give you a place to begin your inquiry.

Age-related macular degeneration

_____

Bone metastases

_____

Fall precautions

_____

Gout

_____

Multiple myeloma

_____

Myelodysplastic syndromes

_____

Neutropenia

_____

Palmar-plantar erythrodysesthesia

_____

Pathological fractures

_____

Secondary hypertension

_____

Stage I pressure ulcer

_____

Thrombocytopenia

_____

A 68-year-old male is admitted from the emergency department after falling at home. He states that he has been fatigued and has severe pain in his pelvic area and back. He was unable to button his shirt or walk normally before the fall, and now he has increased pain and burning in his hands and feet. He wants to stop all his medications.

Home Medications

Allopurinol 300 mg tab orally daily

Clopidogrel (Plavix) 75 mg orally 1 daily

Dexamethasone on Thursdays 4-mg tab orally

Ferrous sulfate 27 mg orally with breakfast

Folic acid 1-mg tab orally daily

Furosemide 40 mg orally daily

Lenalidomide 25-mg capsule with lunch orally daily

Morphine (MSIR) 15 mg sublingually as needed for breakthrough pain

Morphine sulfate controlled-release (MS Contin) 60 mg every 12 hours

Multivitamin 1tab orally daily with copper

Ocuvite 1 tab daily orally

Phenytoin 100 mg daily orally (states that he should take 3 times a day but does not)

Potassium chloride 40 mEq orally daily

Sertraline 25-mg tab orally at bedtime

Simvastatin 20-mg tab orally daily

Warfarin (Coumadin) 1-mg tab orally daily

Self-Query

Using a drug book or pharmacology text that contains the mechanism of action, unlabeled uses, and pharmacokinetics of medications, answer the following questions. Make answers specific to this scenario.

What do I know about these medications? Do I know the recommended dose of, the recommended route for, and the best time of day to give these medications? Do I know what lab results I need regarding each medication? Do I know the approved use of each medication? Do I know the most common diseases treated by the listed medications? Are any off-label uses approved for each drug?

Allopurinol

_____

_____

Clopidogrel

_____

_____

Dexamethasone

_____

_____

Ferrous sulfate

_____

_____

Folic acid

_____

_____

Furosemide

_____

_____

Lenalidomide

_____

_____

Morphine

_____

_____

Morphine sulfate, controlled-release

_____

_____

Multivitamin

_____

_____

Ocuvite

_____

_____

Phenytoin

_____

_____

Potassium chloride

_____

_____

Sertraline

_____

_____

Simvastatin

_____

_____

Warfarin

_____

_____

What do these medications tell me about this man's medical history?

_____

_____

What type of pain is controlled by phenytoin? Would this patient be prone to having this type of pain? Can I name three other reasons that the drug would be used, and the precautions?

_____

_____

_____

What is being treated with the lenalidomide? What classification is lenalidomide? Why is it usually given? In what way is the patient able to receive the medication?

_____

_____

_____

Allergies

Meperidine (Demerol)—caused a seizure

Penicillin (PCN)—caused rash

Colchicine—caused diarrhea, nausea, and vomiting

Self-Query

Do I know the signs and symptoms of an adverse reaction to meperidine? Do I know meperidine's classification? What is the metabolite of meperidine that would have caused the seizure?

_____

_____

Do I know the signs and symptoms of an adverse reaction to penicillin? Do I know penicillin's classification?

_____

_____

Do I know the signs and symptoms of an adverse reaction to colchicine? Do I know colchicine's classification? Do I know why colchicine would have been ordered for this patient?

_____

_____

Body Systems

Self-Query

Be prepared to defend your answers.

Can I place each medication under the body system that it commonly affects?

Neurological

_____

Cardiovascular

_____

Hematological

_____

Pulmonary

_____

Gastrointestinal

_____

Nutrition

_____

Genitourinary/renal

_____

Musculoskeletal

_____

Endocrine

_____

Integumentary

_____

Immune

_____

Pain/comfort

_____

Mechanism of Action

？ Self-Query

Does the individual's medical history have an effect on the pharmacokinetics of each drug?

_____

_____

What contraindications do I need to address regarding the medications and medical history?

_____

_____

Nursing Process

？ Self-Query

What nursing assessment will I perform regarding each medication? What planning and implementation do I need to do regarding each medication? How do I evaluate each medication's effectiveness?

Allopurinol

_____

_____

Clopidogrel

_____

_____

Dexamethasone

_____

_____

Ferrous sulfate

_____

_____

Folic acid

_____

_____

Furosemide

_____

_____

Lenalidomide

_____

_____

Morphine

_____

_____

Morphine sulfate controlled-release

_____

_____

Multivitamin

_____

_____

Ocuvite

_____

_____

Phenytoin

_____

_____

Potassium chloride

_____

_____

Sertraline

_____

_____

Simvastatin

_____

_____

Warfarin

_____

_____

Do I need to be concerned about geriatric considerations for this individual?

_____

_____

Physical Assessment Findings

Neurological Assessment

Pleasant, alert, oriented to time and place

Pupils equal, round, and reactive to light; patient wears glasses

Weakness noted in all extremities

Cardiovascular and Hematological Assessment

K+ 3.5, S_1S_2 monitor reveals sinus of 68

Blood pressure 100/50 no edema, extremities pale, capillary refill at 3 seconds

Bruising to upper extremities and bruising noted on shins bilaterally

History of absolute neutrophil count < 1000

Platelets 175,000; RBC 4.0; Hct 29; Hgb 10; WBC 3000

Pulmonary Assessment

Clear throughout with respiratory rate 16 per minute

O_2 @ 2 L (presently wearing), O_2 sat at 94%

Gastrointestinal Assessment

Oral cavity pale; wears dentures but states that his mouth hurts and he cannot wear them

Has lost 5 pounds in 2 weeks

Genitourinary Assessment

Denies problems

Musculoskeletal Assessment

Noted muscle weakness, unable to stand without assistance

Endocrine Assessment

Labs within normal findings; no outward signs of problems

Integumentary Assessment

Bruising to upper extremities; bruising noted on shins bilaterally

Noted redness and IV site to right antecubital 0.9% NS

Immune Assessment

History of absolute neutrophil count < 1000

Platelets 175,000; RBC 4.0; Hct 29; Hgb 10; WBC 3000

Pain/Comfort Assessment

Burning sensations in hands and feet

Deep aching in hip area

Unable to stand without assistance or button his shirt because of pain

Physician Orders

Complete blood count

INR

Leukocyte alkaline phosphate

? Self-Query

Develop two nursing diagnoses for this patient (NANDA).

_____

_____

Develop at least three patient outcomes (NOC).

_____

_____

_____

Develop at least three patient interventions (NIC).

_____

_____

_____

Synopsis

26

Because you can find answers to the self-queries in numerous texts, you will not find the answers to all of them here. However, you will find discussion of the individual cases. The scenario relates to chemotherapy toxicity; therefore, purposefully look into the medication use and vocabulary as they relate to these factors.

Vocabulary

When reviewing the vocabulary words, you might want to ask several questions: who, what, where, when, why, and how. This should give you a much broader understanding of each word.

Do yourself a favor and do not just give the shortest and simplest answer. Use the following example of multiple myeloma: Instead of answering, "Multiple myeloma is a cancer of the white blood cells," ask:

Who is at risk for **multiple myeloma**? What medications can cause multiple myeloma? What medications can treat it?

☑ Self-Query: Possible Answers

When defining the remainder of the vocabulary words, ask the following questions:

What is **age-related macular degeneration**? How is it treated?

Who is at risk for **bone metastases**? If a person has bone cancer, where does it metastasize to? What medications can treat it?

Why use **fall precautions** in individuals on chemotherapy? How is peripheral neuropathy related to falls?

What is **gout**? Which chemotherapy medications are major contributors to gout? What medications are used to treat it?

What is a **myelodysplastic syndrome**? Who is at risk? What places patients at risk? How is it treated?

What is **neutropenia**? What are neutropenic precautions? How is neutropenia treated with medications?

What is another term for **palmar-plantar erythrodysesthesia**? What are the symptoms? Who is at risk? How is it treated?

What is a **pathological fracture**? Who is at risk? How is it related to chemotherapy in cancer?

What is **secondary hypertension**? Which chemotherapy medications are major contributors to secondary hypertension? What medications are used to treat it?

What is a **stage I pressure ulcer**? What is the treatment? Is it common in cancer patients?

What is **thrombocytopenia**? Are there special precautions? How is thrombocytopenia treated with medications?

Home Medications

Allopurinol 300-mg tab orally daily: increased uric acid in blood (possible gout)

Clopidogrel (Plavix) 75 mg orally 1 daily: possible increased clotting (DVT/TIA)

Dexamethasone on Thursdays 4-mg tab orally: inflammatory response (need for decreased response)

Ferrous sulfate 27 mg orally with breakfast: nutritional deficiency

Folic acid 1-mg tab orally daily: nutritional deficiency

Furosemide 40 mg orally daily: problems with fluid excess (cardiac/hypertension)

Lenalidomide 25-mg capsule with lunch orally daily: used in multiple myeloma; known for causing thromboembolism, particularly when combined with dexamethasone

Morphine (MSIR) 15 mg sublingually as needed for breakthrough pain: severe pain (used between doses of morphine sulfate controlled-release [MS Contin])

Morphine sulfate controlled-release 60 mg every 12 hours: severe pain

Multivitamin 1 tab orally daily with copper: nutritional deficiency

Ocuvite 1 tab daily orally: macular degeneration

Phenytoin 100 mg daily orally (states he should take 3 times a day but doesn't): neurological issues (seizure activity or neuropathic pain)

Potassium chloride 40 mEq orally daily: supplement with diuretic

Sertraline 25-mg tab orally at bedtime: depression (selective serotonin reuptake inhibitor [SSRI])

Simvastatin 20-mg tab orally daily: lowers cholesterol

Warfarin (Coumadin) 1-mg tab orally daily: possible increased clotting (DVT)

Phenytoin is an adjunct medication for neuropathic pain. Chemotherapy medications may damage nerve endings and cause this type of pain. This drug is also used for seizures, cardiac, and dermatology. Common side effects include gingival hyperplasia, blood disorders, and bradycardia.

A note concerning the home meds: The oncologist stated that combining lenalidomide and dexamethasone delayed the progression of advanced multiple myeloma.

Lenalidomide is used for treating multiple myeloma and is known for causing thromboembolism, particularly when combined with dexamethasone. It is a derivative of thalidomide. Under current FDA rules, only individuals who are registered with the RevAssist program can obtain lenalidomide; only healthcare providers who are registered with RevAssist can prescribe it; and only a registered pharmacy can dispense it.

Allergies

✓ Self-Query: Possible Answers

Meperidine (Demerol) is a major opioid analgesic. This individual took oral meperidine for severe pain. Unfortunately, he developed an accumulation of normeperidine, meperidine's metabolite, which caused his seizure. He was prescribed morphine, which does not have the ceiling limit.

An allergy to penicillin (PCN) is not uncommon; many individuals develop an allergic reaction to this antibiotic.

Colchicine is an anti-inflammatory medication given for gout. This is not really an allergy; it is a major side effect of this medication when given orally. Many times, IV administration can alleviate this effect.

Body Systems

☑ Self-Query: Possible Answers

Neurological

> Phenytoin 100 mg daily orally
> Sertraline 25-mg tab orally at bedtime
> Morphine sulfate controlled-release 60 mg every 12 hours
> Morphine 15 mg sublingually as needed for breakthrough pain

Cardiovascular

> None specific; however, phenytoin can alter cardiac function.

Hematological

> Allopurinol 300-mg tab orally daily
> Warfarin 1-mg tab orally daily
> Dexamethasone on Thursdays 4-mg tab orally
> Folic acid 1-mg tab orally daily
> Ferrous sulfate 27 mg orally with breakfast
> Multivitamin 1 tab orally daily with copper
> Clopidogrel 75 mg orally 1 daily
> Potassium chloride 40 mEq orally daily
> Furosemide 40 mg orally daily
> Lenalidomide 25-mg capsule with lunch orally daily
> Simvastatin 20-mg tab orally daily
> Some may also place Ocuvite here

Pulmonary

> None specific

Gastrointestinal

> None specific

Nutrition

> Allopurinol 300-mg tab orally daily
> Folic acid 1-mg tab orally daily
> Ferrous sulfate 27 mg orally with breakfast
> Ocuvite 1 tab daily orally
> Multivitamin 1 tab orally daily with copper
> Simvastatin 20-mg tab orally daily

Genitourinary/renal

> Allopurinol 300-mg tab orally daily
> Potassium chloride 40 mEq orally daily
> Furosemide 40 mg orally daily

Musculoskeletal

> Dexamethasone on Thursdays 4-mg tab orally (not specific for skeletal but can alter bone density)
> Folic acid 1-mg tab orally daily
> Ferrous sulfate 27 mg orally with breakfast
> Multivitamin 1 tab orally daily with copper
> Lenalidomide 25-mg capsule with lunch orally daily

Endocrine

Dexamethasone on Thursdays 4-mg tab orally (not specific for endocrine but can alter glucose
levels)

Integumentary

Not specific for integumentary but can alter skin integrity

Immune

Lenalidomide 25-mg capsule with lunch orally daily (not specific for the immune system but can
affect the body's ability to fight infection)

Pain/comfort

Phenytoin 100 mg daily orally
Sertraline 25-mg tab orally at bedtime
Morphine sulfate controlled-release 60 mg every 12 hours
Morphine 15 mg sublingually as needed for breakthrough pain

Physician Orders

☑ Self-Queries: Possible Answers

This gentleman was diagnosed with peripheral neuropathy. It was apparent from the medication list
he brought from home that this was not a new issue for him. An MRI was added to the requests. The
patient not only had increased peripheral neuropathy from the fall (caused by the neuropathy in his feet)
but also had fractured his hip. In addition, he had spinal cord compression. He underwent a percutaneous vertebroplasty, which gave him moderate relief. Major spinal surgery was not a practical treatment
option. Teaching should include ways to decrease the pain caused by the neuropathy.

Case Study Inquiry

27

Vocabulary

☞ Self-Query

Before attempting to work the case study, define each of the vocabulary words. Although the words may have several subheadings, it will give you a place to begin your inquiry.

Antibacterial
_____

Antifungal
_____

Anti-infectives
_____

Cephalosporin
_____

Community-associated MRSA
_____

Fluoroquinolones
_____

Healthcare-associated MRSA
_____

Long-term care facility
_____

Staphylococcus aureus
_____

Staphylococcus epidermidis
_____

Staphylococcus pneumonia
_____

Suprainfection
_____

The patient, a 54-year-old female, is a cafeteria worker in a local middle school. She states that last week she developed a red raised area on her right thigh. She states that she thought it was a pimple. It was sore, so she covered it with a large bandage and today presents with a 2 cm × 2 cm red open area that is tender and warm to touch. It is also draining thick green pus. She has a fever of 101°F. Small blisters are spreading to other areas.

Physician Orders

Culture and sensitivity of drainage to right thigh

Blood cultures

IV linezolid 600 mg now, and admit to medical floor for possible wound drainage

? Self-Query

What classification is linezolid? Why is it usually given? How is it given? Do I know why the physician ordered it for this individual? What side effects should be expected for this person?

Home Medications

Medication reconciliation is performed before sending patient to the medical unit.

Acetaminophen (Tylenol) ES 1–2 capsules every 4 hours as needed for headache or fever

Calcium citrate (Citracal) 250 with vitamin D, 1 tab daily

Docusate 100 mg twice a day

Hydroxychloroquine sulfate (Plaquenil) 200 mg orally twice a day

Ibuprofen (Motrin) 800 mg orally every 12 hours as needed for joint pain

Methotrexate 7.5 mg orally every Monday

Nebivolol (Bystolic) 5 mg orally daily

Paroxetine (Paxil) 20 mg orally at bedtime

Rabeprazole sodium (AcipHex) 20 mg orally daily

? Self-Query

Using a drug book or pharmacology text that contains the mechanism of action, unlabeled uses, and pharmacokinetics for medications, answer the following questions. Make answers specific to this scenario.

What do I know about these medications? Do I know the recommended dose of, the recommended route for, and the best time of day to give these medications? Do I know what lab results I need regarding each medication? Do I know the approved use of each medication? Do I know the most common diseases treated by the listed medications? Are any off-label uses approved for each drug?

Acetaminophen

_____

_____

Calcium citrate

_____

_____

Docusate

_____

_____

Hydroxychloroquine sulfate

_____

_____

Ibuprofen

_____

_____

Methotrexate

_____

_____

Nebivolol

_____

_____

Paroxetine

_____

_____

Rabeprazole sodium

_____

_____

What do these medications tell me about this patient's health history?

_____

_____

How would the patient's immune system be affected by the medications?

_____

_____

Can I name the medications most likely to affect the immune system?

_____

Do I know which medications the physician will place on hold?

_____

Allergies

Infliximab

? Self-Query

Do I know the signs and symptoms of an adverse reaction to infliximab? Do I know infliximab's classification? What is infliximab's brand name? Why was infliximab ordered for this patient?

_____

_____

Body Systems

? Self-Query

Be prepared to defend your answers.

Can I place each medication under the body system that it commonly affects?

Neurological

_____

Cardiovascular

_____

Hematological

_____

Pulmonary

_____

Gastrointestinal

_____

Nutrition

_____

Genitourinary/renal

_____

Musculoskeletal

_____

Endocrine

_____

Integumentary

_____

Immune

_____

Pain/comfort

_____

Mechanism of Action

? Self-Query

Does the individual's medical history have an effect on the pharmacokinetics of each drug?

_____

_____

What contraindications do I need to address regarding the medications and medical history?

_____

_____

Nursing Process

? Self-Query

What nursing assessment will I perform regarding each medication? What planning and implementation do I need to do in regard to each medication? How do I evaluate each medication's effectiveness?

Acetaminophen

_____

_____

Calcium citrate

_____

_____

Docusate

_____

_____

Hydroxychloroquine sulfate

_____

_____

Ibuprofen

_____

_____

Methotrexate

_____

_____

Nebivolol

_____

_____

Paroxetine

_____

_____

Rabeprazole sodium

_____

_____

The culture and sensitivity returns and the report reveals c-susceptible staph (methicillin-susceptible *Staphylococcus aureus*). Can the patient remain on the linezolid?

_____

_____

Is the medication linezolid appropriate for the bacteria?

_____

_____

Develop two nursing diagnoses for this patient (NANDA).

_____

_____

Develop at least three patient outcomes (NOC).

_____

_____

_____

Develop at least three patient interventions (NIC).

_____

_____

_____

Synopsis

27

Because you can find answers to the self-queries in numerous texts, you will not find the answers to all of them here. However, you will find discussion of the individual case. The scenario relates to methicillin-resistant staph complications; therefore, purposefully look into the medication use and vocabulary as they relate to these factors.

Vocabulary

When reviewing the vocabulary words, you might want to ask several questions: who, what, where, when, why, and how. This should give you a much broader understanding of each word.

Do yourself a favor and do not just give the shortest and simplest answer. Use the following example of prostaglandins: Instead of answering, "Community-associated MRSA is an infection acquired in the community," ask:

Who is at risk for **community-associated MRSA**? What is the treatment for community-associated MRSA?

☑ Self-Query: Possible Answers

When defining the remainder of the vocabulary words, ask the following questions:

What makes a medication **antibacterial**? What is the difference between a bacteriostatic and an antibacterial? What determines the difference?

What is an **antifungal**? How are these mediations used? What is the difference between an antifungal and an antibacterial?

What medications are considered **anti-infectives**?

What is a **cephalosporin**? When are they used?

What are **fluoroquinolones**? When are they used?

Who is at risk for **healthcare-associated MRSA**? What is the difference between community-associated MRSA and healthcare-associated MRSA?

What is the definition of a **long-term care facility**? Who lives in a long-term care facility? What are the main criteria for admission?

What is *Staphylococcus epidermidis*? How can it be dangerous?

What is *Staphylococcus aureus*? How can it be dangerous?

What is *Staphylococcus pneumonia*? Who is at risk? How is it treated?

What causes a **suprainfection**? Who is at risk?

Physician Orders

☑ Self-Query: Possible Answers

Linezolid is an oxazolidinone antibiotic; it is active against most gram-positive bacteria, those known to cause MRSA. It has no significant effect on most gram-negative bacteria, so if it is prescribed and does not have an effect, another medication needs to be ordered. The culture has to be obtained before the medication is given. It can be given orally or by IV. The physician suspected MRSA because of the patient's medical history.

Home Medications

☑ Self-Query: Possible Answers

Acetaminophen (Tylenol) ES 1–2 capsules every 4 hours as needed for headache or fever: mild to moderate pain

Calcium citrate (Citracal) 250 with Vitamin D, 1 tab daily: the patient's age places her at risk for osteoarthritis. Many women have low calcium and vitamin D intake, which places them at risk for osteoporosis.

Docusate 100 mg twice a day: self-medication for constipation

Hydroxychloroquine sulfate (Plaquenil) 200 mg orally twice a day: can be prescribed for the prevention and treatment of certain forms of malaria. However, in this case, it was prescribed for the treatment of rheumatoid arthritis (RA). It can also be prescribed for lupus.

Ibuprofen (Motrin) 800 mg orally every 12 hours as needed for joint pain: NSAID used for pain

Methotrexate 7.5 mg orally every Monday: used in certain cancer treatments. It is also most effective in treating various forms of arthritis and other rheumatic conditions. It is classified here as a disease-modifying antirheumatic drug (DMARD). The major oral complication is nausea.

Nebivolol (Bystolic) 5 mg orally daily: beta-blocker, used to treat hypertension

Paroxetine (Paxil) 20 mg orally at bedtime: depression (SSRI)

Rabeprazole sodium (AcipHex) 20 mg orally daily: decreases the amount of acid produced in the stomach.

Allergies

☑ Self-Query: Possible Answers

Because infliximab (Remicade) is an infusion medication, the reports of allergy usually occur during, or within a few hours of, the infusion. Signs of an adverse reaction are fever, chills chest pain, and hypo- or hypertension. Be aware that infliximab alters the immune system and lowers the body's ability to fight infection. Infliximab blocks the production of the tumor necrosis factor-alpha (TNF-alpha). TNF-alpha is made by the body's immune system. Infliximab was ordered for this patient because it works for any autoimmune disease—in this case, RA. Infliximab was prescribed was prescribed along with methotrexate, which the individual is still receiving, works to reduce the progression of structural damage and therefore limits damage from severe RA.

Body Systems

☑ Self-Query: Possible Answers

Neurological

Paroxetine 20 mg orally at bedtime

Cardiovascular

Nebivolol 5 mg orally daily

Hematological

Hydroxychloroquine sulfate 200 mg orally twice a day
Methotrexate 7.5 mg orally every Monday

Pulmonary

None specific

Gastrointestinal

Rabeprazole sodium 20 mg orally daily
Calcium citrate 250 with vitamin D 1 tab daily
Docusate 100 mg twice a day
Some may have placed MTX here because of its effect on this system.

Nutrition

Calcium citrate 250 with vitamin D, 1 tab daily

Genitourinary/renal

None specific

Musculoskeletal

Hydroxychloroquine sulfate 200 mg orally twice a day
Methotrexate 7.5 mg orally every Monday
Acetaminophen ES 1–2 capsules every 4 hours as needed for headache or fever
Ibuprofen 800 mg orally every 12 hours as needed for joint pain
Calcium citrate 250 with vitamin D, 1 tab daily

Endocrine

None specific

Integumentary

IV linezolid 600 mg is placed here because of a skin infection.

Immune

Hydroxychloroquine sulfate 200 mg orally twice a day
Methotrexate 7.5 mg orally every Monday
Most individuals take it on a weekend day. This patient chose Monday so that she would better
    remember to take it.

Pain/comfort

Acetaminophen ES 1–2 capsules every 4 hours as needed for headache or fever
Ibuprofen 800 mg orally every 12 hours as needed for joint pain

Be aware that the medications she is taking to decrease the RA symptoms are considered pain and
comfort medications.

Nursing Process

☑ Self-Query: Possible Answers

The patient could remain on linezolid once the culture and sensitivity report revealed methicillin-susceptible staph aureus, but the physician changed the therapy to nafcillin. She was monitored closely to assess for emerging resistance.

Just a note: The contact with the bacteria would probably not have been an issue if her immune system was not altered by her medications. Additionally, she had received infliximab several times before she developed the infusion reaction. Her immune system was compromised; however, her medications allowed her to continue working at a job she has held for 25 years.

Case Study Inquiry

28

Vocabulary

Self-Query

Before attempting to work the case study, define each of the vocabulary words. Although the words may have several subheadings, it will give you a place to begin your inquiry.

Asbestosis

_____

COPD

_____

Cor pulmonale

_____

C-reactive protein

_____

Extravasation of vesicant

_____

Giant cell lung cancer

_____

Lymph nodes

_____

Oat cell carcinoma

_____

Spinal stenosis

_____

Telomere

_____

Recent History

After being diagnosed with Stage IV non-small cell lung cancer in 2008, your 64-year-old female patient requested to enroll in a genomics-guided lung cancer treatment protocol. It was available only in North Carolina, so she had to travel and remain there until the chemo cycles were complete. The genomic analysis determined that her tumor was resistant to cisplatin, a commonly used front-line chemotherapy drug, so she was treated with a combination of pemetrexed and gemcitabine. Now she has returned home for a follow-up with her local oncologist. The oncologist discussed the fact that the results from a recent exam revealed that "the size of tumor has shrunk by more than 60 percent."

What is the classification of these medications? What is the trade name of these medications? Which cell cycle phase is affected? What is its most common dose-limiting toxicity? What routes can be used to administer this medication?

Cisplatin

_____

_____

Pemetrexed

_____

_____

Gemcitabine

_____

_____

Home Medications

Albuterol (Proventil) 2.5 mg/3 mL (0.083% nebulizer solution) 2.5 mg every 4–6 hours

Esomeprazole (Nexium) 40 mg orally before lunch

Furosemide (Lasix) 40 mg orally before breakfast

Insulin glargine (Lantus) 40 units subcutaneously at bedtime

Nebivolol (Bystolic) 5 mg orally daily

Potassium chloride (K-Dur) 20 mEq taken with furosemide

Prednisone 5 mg orally daily

Theophylline (Slo-Bid) 200 mg orally twice a day (every 12 hours)

Tramadol (Ultram) 100 mg extended release daily

Self-Query

Using a drug book or pharmacology text that contains the mechanism of action, unlabeled uses, and pharmacokinetics for medications, answer the following questions. Make answers specific to this scenario.

What do I know about these medications? Do I know the recommended dose of, the recommended route for, and the best time of day to give these medications? Do I know what lab results I need regarding each medication? Do I know the approved use of each medication? Do I know the most common diseases treated by the listed medications? Are any off-label uses approved for each drug?

Albuterol

_____

_____

Esomeprazole

_____

_____

Furosemide

_____

Insulin glargine

_____

_____

Nebivolol

_____

_____

Potassium chloride

_____

_____

Prednisone

_____

_____

Theophylline

_____

_____

Tramadol

_____

_____

Do I know the individual's past medical history by looking at the medication list?

Allergies

Ciprofloxacin (Cipro)

Self-Query

Do I know why Cipro would have been prescribed? Do I know what other drugs are in Cipro's classification? Do I know the signs and symptoms of an adverse reaction to Cipro? Do I know how this drug works?

_____

_____

How does Cipro interact with theophylline? Is the patient currently taking theophylline?

_____

_____

Body Systems

Self-Query

Be prepared to defend your answers.

Can I place each medication under the body system that it commonly affects?

Neurological

_____

Cardiovascular

_____

Hematological

_____

Pulmonary

_____

Gastrointestinal

_____

Nutrition

_____

Genitourinary/renal

_____

Musculoskeletal

_____

Endocrine

_____

Integumentary

_____

Immune

_____

Pain/comfort

_____

Mechanism of Action

? Self-Query

Are there any factors in the individual's medical history that may affect the pharmacokinetics of each drug?

_____

_____

What contraindications do I need to address regarding the medications and medical history?

_____

_____

Nursing Process

? Self-Query

What nursing assessment will I perform for each medication? What planning and implementation do I need to do in regard to each medication? How do I evaluate each medication's effectiveness?

Albuterol

_____

_____

Cisplatin

_____

_____

Esomeprazole

_____

_____

Furosemide

_____

_____

Gemcitabine

_____

_____

Insulin glargine

_____

_____

Nebivolol

_____

_____

Pemetrexed

_____

_____

Potassium chloride

_____

_____

Prednisone

_____

_____

Theophylline

_____

_____

Tramadol

_____

_____

Synopsis

28

Because you can find answers to the self-queries in numerous texts, you will not find the answers to all of them here. However, you will find discussion of the individual cases. The scenario relates to chemotherapy and genomics; therefore, purposefully look into the medication use and vocabulary as they relate to these factors.

Vocabulary

When reviewing the vocabulary words, you might want to ask several questions: who, what, where, when, why, and how. This should give you a much broader understanding of each word.

Do yourself a favor and do not just give the shortest and simplest answer. Use the following example of COPD: Instead of answering, "COPD is a lung disease," ask:

Who develops **COPD**? What are the major causes of COPD? What medications treat COPD?

☑ Self-Query: Possible Answers

When defining the remainder of the vocabulary words, ask the following questions:

What is **asbestosis**? Who is at risk for asbestosis? What medications treat asbestosis?

What is **cor pulmonale**? What are the major causes of cor pulmonale? What medications treat cor pulmonale?

What is the **C-reactive protein**? What can it tell us?

What does **extravasation of vesicant** cause? What medications are considered vesicants? Why would this individual be receiving a vesicant?

What is **giant cell lung cancer**? Which medications treat it?

Where are **lymph nodes** located? What is their function?

What is **oat cell carcinoma**? Which medications treat it?

What is **spinal stenosis**? Who is at risk for spinal stenosis?

What is a **telomere**? Where are they located? Why are they important?

Recent History

☑ Self-Query: Possible Answers

Cisplatin (Platinol) is a platinum-based cancer drug. It is an alkylating drug and works in the resting phase of the cell. It alters tumor cells by stopping reproduction of DNA and interfering with the reproduction of cells. It is cell-cycle nonspecific. The most common side effects are nausea and vomiting, renal toxicity, anemia, and neutropenia. It is always given as an infusion. Note to yourself what is and what is not IV compatible.

Pemetrexed (Alimta) is an IV medication known as a folate antimetabolite. Methotrexate is also in this category. It disrupts the metabolic process that is dependent on folate for cell reproduction. Because it alters folate, the individual administered this medication needs take folate and B12 supplements to protect the stomach, blood cells, and bone marrow.

Gemcitabine (Gemzar) is an IV medication known as an antimetabolite. It replaces one of the building blocks of nucleic acid, thus interfering with DNA replication. One of the most common alterations is myelosuppression. It is administered over 30 minutes via IV.

Allergies

☑ Self-Query: Possible Answers

Ciprofloxacin (Cipro) is fluoroquinolone antibiotic. It destroys bacteria by interfering with DNA duplication. One adverse reaction is a rash. However, this individual reported severe joint and muscle pain. Ciprofloxacin may increase the serum concentrations of theophylline. Ciprofloxacin inhibits the metabolism of theophylline in the liver, which creates theophylline toxicity.

Body Systems

☑ Self-Query: Possible Answers

Neurological

Tramadol (Ultram) 100 mg extended release daily

Cardiovascular

Furosemide (Lasix) 40 mg orally before breakfast
Potassium chloride (K-Dur) 20 mEq taken with furosemide
Nebivolol (Bystolic) 5 mg orally daily

Hematological

Furosemide 40 mg orally before breakfast
Potassium chloride 20 mEq taken with furosemide
Prednisone 5 mg orally daily

Pulmonary

Theophylline (Slo-Bid) 200 mg orally twice a day (every 12 hours)
Prednisone 5 mg orally daily
Albuterol (Proventil) 2.5 mg/3 mL (0.083% nebulizer solution) 2.5 mg

Gastrointestinal

Esomeprazole (Nexium) 40 mg orally before lunch

Nutrition

None specific

Genitourinary/renal

Furosemide 40 mg orally before breakfast
Potassium chloride 20 mEq taken with furosemide

Musculoskeletal

Tramadol 100 mg extended release daily

Endocrine

Prednisone 5 mg orally daily (will alter glucose metabolism)
Insulin glargine (Lantus) 40 units subcutaneously at bedtime

Integumentary

Prednisone 5 mg orally daily (will alter skin integrity)

Immune

Prednisone 5 mg orally daily (will decrease the body's ability to fight infection)

Pain/comfort

Tramadol 100 mg extended release daily

Nursing Process

☑ Self-Query: Possible Answers

Group discussion is on the genomics used to treat this individual.

Note: The patient also took folate and B12 on a daily schedule to alter the possible side effects of the folate antimetabolites, pemetrexed (Alimta).

Case Study Inquiry

29

Before attempting to work the case study, define each of the vocabulary words. Although the words may have several subheadings, it will give you a place to begin your inquiry.

Vocabulary

❓ Self-Query

Alcoholic hepatitis

_____

Ascites

_____

Asterixis

_____

Cirrhosis

_____

Esophageal varices

_____

Hepatic encephalopathy

_____

Hepatitis

_____

Liver cancer

_____

Multiple myeloma

_____

Paracentesis

_____

Portal hypertension

_____

Spontaneous bacterial peritonitis

_____

A 65-year-old male patient has been admitted to the medical floor for an abdominal paracentesis. He arrived at the emergency room with severe abdominal and respiratory distress.

Home Medications

Aspirin (Ecotrin) as needed for headache and joint pain

Furosemide (Lasix) 80 mg every 12 hours orally

Insulin glargine (Lantus) 30 units subcutaneously at bedtime

Lactulose (Cephulac) when needed

Omeprazole 20 mg orally with breakfast and lunch

Pancrelipase 2-unit capsules with meals (breakfast, lunch, and dinner)

Potassium chloride (KCl) 40 mg every 12 hours orally

Regular insulin 3 units subcutaneously with breakfast and dinner

Thalidomide 50 mg orally 2 capsules at bedtime

Self-Query

Using a drug book or pharmacology text that contains the mechanism of action, unlabeled uses, and pharmacokinetics for medications, answer the following questions. Make answers specific to this scenario.

What do I know about these medications? Do I know the recommended dose of, the recommended route for, and the best time of day to give these medications? Do I know what lab results I need regarding each medication? Do I know the approved use of each medication? Do I know the most common diseases treated by the listed medications? Are any off-label uses approved for each drug?

Aspirin

_____

_____

Furosemide

_____

_____

Insulin glargine

_____

_____

Lactulose

_____

_____

Omeprazole

_____

_____

Pancrelipase

_____

_____

Potassium chloride

_____

_____

Regular insulin

_____

_____

Thalidomide

_____

_____

Do I know the individual's past medical history by looking at the medication list?

_____

_____

Body Systems

Be prepared to defend your answers.

Self-Query

Can I place each medication under the body system that it commonly affects?

Neurological
_____

Cardiovascular
_____

Hematological
_____

Pulmonary
_____

Gastrointestinal
_____

Nutrition
_____

Genitourinary/renal
_____

Musculoskeletal
_____

Endocrine
_____

Integumentary
_____

Immune
_____

Pain/comfort
_____

Physical Assessment Findings
Neurological Assessment

Acute confusion and slurred speech, noted lethargy

Asterixis noted

Cardiovascular and Hematological Assessment

Ascites noted INR: 5 and the K+2.9

Cardiac enlargement noted on CXR

Blood pressure 200/110, dependent edema, extremities jaundiced

Noted bruising to upper extremities and on shins bilaterally

Pulmonary Assessment

Respiratory rate is 12

Clubbing is noted

Dyspnea is noted even while on 4 liters of oxygen

Auscultation reveals crackles throughout lung fields

Gastrointestinal Assessment

Hyperactive bowel sounds, fetor hepaticus noted, poor dentations

Patient's wife states no bowel movement for 4 days

Large distended abdominal girth

Nausea

AST/ALT normal at this time; has been extremely elevated: ALP 130

Elevated bilirubin

Genitourinary Assessment

Foley inserted, 100 mL dark (tea-colored) urine returned

Musculoskeletal Assessment

Noted tenderness to hands and feet

Restricted ability to coordinate movements

Endocrine Assessment

Elevated aldosterone level

Elevated cortisol level

Integumentary Assessment

Noted bruising to upper extremities and on shins bilaterally

Severe red, flaky patches of dry skin

IV site to right antecubital 0.9% NS

Immune Assessment

No palpable lymph nodes, WBC: 2.5

Pain/Comfort Assessment

Grimace during abdominal palpation and measuring girth

Noted scratch marks on extremity (patient states dry and itching)

Physician Orders

Schedule paracentesis:

Albumin 25% undiluted 200 mL infused during paracentesis and daily

Stop:

Thalidomide
Aspirin

Start:

Lactulose 10 gram/15 mL; 50 mL syrup every 6 hours for three bowel movements
Ammonium lactate topical (Lac-Hydrin) 12% cream, apply thin layer to extremities
Omeprazole 20 mg orally with breakfast and lunch
Mirtazapine (Remeron) 30-mg tab orally at bedtime

Nursing Process

Self-Query

Without consulting a pharmacology text, what do I already know about these medications?

_____

_____

What is the whole picture, considering both old and new medications?

_____

_____

For each medication, do I know the recommended dose, the recommended route, and the best time of day to give it? Do I know what lab results I need in regard to each medication? Are any off-label uses approved for each drug?

Ammonium lactate topical

_____

_____

Mirtazapine

_____

_____

The patient's wife asks why some of his medications have been changed. She thought the aspirin could be used because it is enteric coated. What information does she need?

_____

_____

You remember hearing that thalidomide is an older medication and that it was unavailable in the United States until the late 1990s. Why would this patient be taking thalidomide? Why was this medication restricted?

_____

_____

After you speak with the patient and his wife, they decide they want to go to hospice. What medications are available on hospice, and who will pay for them?

_____

_____

Synopsis

29

Because you can find answers to the self-queries in numerous texts, you will not find the answers to all of them here. However, you will find discussion of the individual case. The scenario relates to cirrhosis medications; therefore, purposefully look into the medication use and vocabulary as they relate to these factors.

Vocabulary

When reviewing the vocabulary words, you might want to ask several questions: who, what, where, when, why, and how. This should give you a much broader understanding of each word.

Do yourself a favor and do not just give the shortest and simplest answer. Use the following example of cirrhosis: Instead of answering, "Cirrhosis is a disease that alters the liver," ask:

Who is at risk for **cirrhosis**? What are its causes? How do medications contribute to cirrhosis?

☑ Self-Query: Possible Answers

When defining the remainder of the vocabulary words, ask the following questions:

What is **alcoholic hepatitis**? How is it treated?

What is **ascites**? What are its causes? How is it treated?

What is **asterixis**? Who is at risk? How is it treated?

What are **esophageal varices**? How do they develop? How are they treated?

What is **hepatic encephalopathy**? What causes it?

What is **hepatitis**? What distinguishes the different types? How are they treated?

What is the major cause of **liver cancer**?

What is **multiple myeloma**?

What is **portal hypertension**? What causes it? What medications treat it?

Why is a **paracentesis** performed? Why is it needed?

What is **spontaneous bacterial peritonitis**?

Home Medications

☑ Self-Queries: Possible Answers

Furosemide (Lasix) 80 mg every 12 hours orally: edema/hypertension

Potassium chloride (KCl) 40 mg every 12 hours orally: electrolyte replacement (on furosemide)

Aspirin (Ecotrin) as needed for headache and joint pain: pain (Note that this medication is enteric coasted and will be altered in the small intestine, not the stomach.)

Thalidomide 50 mg orally 2 capsules at bedtime: approved for use in multiple myeloma

Pancrelipase 2-unit capsules with meals (breakfast, lunch, and dinner): pancreatic lipase is a water-soluble enzyme secreted by the pancreas. It works to break down fats in the intestines. The patient's pancreas is no longer functioning, so he needs supplements.

Insulin glargine (Lantus) 30 units subcutaneously at bedtime: glucose regulation; the patient's pancreas is no longer functioning.

Regular insulin 3 units subcutaneously with breakfast and dinner: glucose regulation; his pancreas is no longer functioning.

Omeprazole 20 mg orally with breakfast and lunch: gastric/esophageal irritation

Lactulose (Cephulac) when needed: used to treat chronic constipation and to treat and prevent complications of liver disease (hepatic encephalopathy).

Body Systems

☑ Self-Queries: Possible Answers

Neurological

> Lactulose when needed
> Yes, it is for constipation; however, when the individual develops hepatic encephalopathy this medication enhances excretion of ammonia.

Cardiovascular

> Furosemide 80 mg every 12 hours orally
> Potassium chloride 40 mg every 12 hours orally

Hematological

> Potassium chloride 40 mg every 12 hours orally
> Thalidomide 50 mg orally 2 capsules at bedtime
> Pancrelipase 2 unit capsules with meals

Gastrointestinal

> Potassium chloride 40 mg every 12 hours orally
> Aspirin as needed (given for pain, but alters GI mucosa)
> Pancrelipase 2-unit capsules with meals
> Lactulose when needed

Nutrition

> Pancrelipase 2-unit capsules with meals
> Insulin glargine 30 units subcutaneously at bedtime
> Regular insulin 3 units subcutaneously with breakfast and dinner

Genitourinary/renal

> Furosemide 80 mg every 12 hours orally
> Potassium chloride 40 mg every 12 hours orally
> Aspirin (given for pain but alters renal profusion by way of prostaglandins)

Musculoskeletal

> Aspirin as needed for headache and joint pain

Endocrine

> Remember that the pancreas is an endocrine and exocrine gland; therefore, both of these functions must be covered when it is impaired.
> Pancrelipase 2-unit capsules with meals

Insulin glargine 30 units subcutaneously at bedtime
Regular insulin 3 units subcutaneously with breakfast and dinner

Integumentary

Furosemide 80 mg every 12 hours orally (fluid excess related to ascites can alter skin integrity)
Thalidomide 50 mg orally 2 capsules at bedtime
Pancrelipase 2-unit capsules with meals (breakfast, lunch, and dinner)

Immune

Thalidomide 50 mg orally 2 capsules at bedtime

Physical Assessment

☑ Self-Query: Possible Answers

Most of the patient's systems were altered.

Physician Orders

☑ Self-Query: Possible Answers

Paracentesis: Physician expected more than 5 liters to be removed. The purpose of infusing the albumin is to avoid intravascular fluid shift and renal failure after a large-volume paracentesis.

Ammonium lactate topical (Lac-Hydrin) is started because it is particularly indicated for the treatment of this individual's type of dry, scaly skin (xerosis).

Mirtazapine (Remeron) is started because it is a tetracyclic antidepressant and is used as a hypnotic.

Nursing Process

☑ Self-Queries: Possible Answers

Explain to the patient's wife that Ecotrin is not effective in his pain management; it is still aspirin, and it alters kidney function and his clotting factors.

Thalidomide was known for causing major birth defects. It was not allowed in the United States of its original use. However, with stringent guidelines, it is currently used in the treatment of certain cancers.

Hospice is an excellent decision for this individual because it includes the whole family in the treatment plan. Medicare and Medicaid have benefit provisions, and numerous private insurance plans have per diem benefits. Most medications related to a hospice diagnosis are covered in the per diem plan.

Case Study Inquiry

30

Vocabulary

Self-Query

Before attempting to work the case study, define each of the vocabulary words. Although the words may have several subheadings, it will give you a place to begin your inquiry.

Alpha cells

_____

Dopamine receptors

_____

Monoamine oxidase inhibitors (MAOIs)

_____

Norepinephrine receptors

_____

Pancreatic beta cells

_____

Pancreatic cells

_____

Pernicious anemia

_____

Serotonin receptors

_____

Vertigo

_____

After attending her sister's wedding reception, a 35-year-old female was admitted for sudden onset of headache, HR 120, nausea and vomiting, and blood pressure of 200/110. During the assessment, the patient cried and said, "I finally felt unafraid to leave the house and ended up screwing up my diet."

Home Medications

Hydrochlorothiazide (HCTZ) 25 mg orally daily

Losartan (Cozaar) 50 mg orally daily

Phenelzine (Nardil) 15 mg orally daily, started 4 weeks ago

Sitagliptin (Januvia) 25 mg orally daily used with diet modifications

Using a drug book or pharmacology text that contains the mechanism of action, unlabeled uses, and pharmacokinetics of medications, answer the following questions. Make answers specific to this scenario.

What do I know about these medications? Do I know the recommended dose of, the recommended route for, and the best time of day to give these medications? Do I know what lab results I need regarding each medication? Do I know the approved use of each medication? Do I know the most common diseases treated by the listed medications? Are any off-label uses approved for each drug?

Hydrochlorothiazide

_____

_____

Losartan

_____

_____

Phenelzine

_____

_____

Sitagliptin

_____

_____

Looking at the medications, what could she mean by her statement?

_____

_____

Do I have an idea of what the patient's medical history might be?

_____

_____

What combination medication could be used instead of the losartan and hydrochlorothiazide?

_____

What are the dangers of using phenelzine?

_____

Nursing Process

? Self-Query

Develop a teaching plan for the patient regarding her home medications.

_____

_____

Develop two nursing diagnoses for this patient (NANDA).

_____

_____

Develop at least three patient outcomes (NOC).

_____

_____

_____

Develop at least three patient interventions (NIC).

_____

_____

_____

Synopsis

30

Because you can find answers to the self-queries in numerous texts, you will not find the answers to all of them here. However, you will find discussion of the individual case. The scenario relates to antidepressant medication-induced hypertension; therefore, purposefully look into the medication use and vocabulary as they relate to these factors.

Vocabulary

When reviewing the vocabulary words, you might want to ask several questions: who, what, where, when, why, and how. This should give you a much broader understanding of each word.

Do yourself a favor and do not just give the shortest and simplest answer. Use the following example of vertigo: Instead of answering, "Vertigo is the feeling of the room spinning," ask:

What causes **vertigo**? Who is at risk for vertigo?

☑ Self-Query: Possible Answers

When defining the remainder of the vocabulary words, ask the following questions:

Where are **alpha cells** located? Which medications alter alpha cells?

What are **dopamine receptors**? Where are they located? Which medications alter them?

What are **monoamine oxidase inhibitors (MAOIs)**? Where is monoamine oxidase located? Who needs it inhibited?

What are **norepinephrine receptors**? Where are they located? Which medications alter them?

Where are **pancreatic beta cells**? Which medications alter beta cells?

What are **pancreatic cells**? How are they endocrine? How are they exocrine?

What is **pernicious anemia**? Who is at risk?

What are **serotonin receptors**? Where are they located? Which medications alter them?

Home Medications

☑ Self-Query: Possible Answers

Hydrochlorothiazide (HCTZ) 25 mg orally daily: hypertension—a diuretic that increases the output of urine; it removes excessive fluid from the cardiovascular system, thus lowering blood pressure.

Losartan (Cozaar) 50 mg orally daily: hypertension—losartan works by preventing the hormone angiotensin II from constricting the blood vessels.

Phenelzine (Nardil) 15 mg orally daily, started 4 weeks ago: it is an MAOI used as an antidepressant in this case. MAO breaks down tyramine, and MAO inhibitors stop this catabolism. Tyramine is found in many drugs, foods, and beverages. If tyramine is not catabolized, a potentially life-threatening rise in blood pressure can occur. Phenelzine, being an MAOI, can cause life-threatening hypertension. The diet that the patient refers to is the one related to phenelzine, not the one related to her type II diabetes. When questioned, the patient said that she had consumed wine and cheeses, and other foods containing tyramine.

Sitagliptin (Januvia) 25 mg orally daily used with diet modifications: type II diabetes—the medication promotes the secretion of insulin by the pancreas and additionally suppresses the release of glucagon by the pancreas.

Hyzaar is a combination medication of losartan and hydrochlorothiazide. The patient had a long history of depression and had been prescribed several antidepressants; phenelzine worked. Because she is now more educated on the side effects of the medication phenelzine, she should be encouraged to return to the use of the medication because it should work without major side effects if the proper diet is followed.

Case Study Inquiry

31

Vocabulary

Self-Query

Before attempting to work the case study, define each of the vocabulary words. Although the words may have several subheadings, it will give you a place to begin your inquiry.

Alpha cells

_____

Anticholinergic effect

_____

Corticosteroids

_____

Dopamine receptors

_____

Folic acid

_____

Hypochromic anemia

_____

Megaloblastic anemia

_____

Norepinephrine receptors

_____

Serotonin receptors

_____

Tyramine

_____

Urushiol

_____

Vertigo

_____

A 61-year-old female is in the office today for a rash from poison ivy that she contacted while working in her backyard. The rash covers her arms and is raised with blisters. She also has a few blisters on her face near her eyes. One of the areas on her arm has a pus formation. She says that she bathed in oatmeal, but the rash does not seem to want to go away.

Home Medications

Aspirin (ASA) 81 mg with breakfast daily

Glyburide 5 mg every 12 hours

Hydrochlorothiazide and losartan (Hyzaar) 50/12.5, 1 tab orally daily

Nortriptyline (Pamelor) 20 mg at bedtime

Sertraline (Zoloft) 50 mg orally daily

Self-Query

Using a drug book or pharmacology text that contains the mechanism of action, unlabeled uses, and pharmacokinetics of medications, answer the following questions. Make answers specific to this scenario.

What do I know about these medications? Do I know the recommended dose of, the recommended route for, and the best time of day to give these medications? Do I know what lab results I need regarding each medication? Do I know the approved use of each medication? Do I know the most common diseases treated by the listed medications? Are any off-label uses approved for each drug?

Aspirin

_____

_____

Glyburide

_____

_____

Hydrochlorothiazide and losartan

_____

_____

Nortriptyline

_____

_____

Sertraline

_____

_____

Nursing Process

Self-Query

What nursing assessment should be performed regarding each medication? What planning and implementation do I need to do regarding each medication? How do I evaluate each medication's effectiveness?

Aspirin

_____

_____

Glyburide

_____

_____

Hydrochlorothiazide and losartan

_____

_____

Nortriptyline

_____

_____

Sertraline

_____

_____

The patient wanted to take Benadryl but was told never to buy anything over the counter without first checking with the office. What is Benadryl's classification? What is its mechanism of action? How would Benadryl affect each of her other medications?

_____

_____

Physician Orders

The FNP prescribes the following medications:

Azithromycin (Zithromax Z-Pak) 500 mg day 1, then 250 mg days 2–5

Prednisone dose pack

The patient is instructed to shower (not bathe) in hot water with antibacterial soap, to take an oatmeal bath (OTC purchase) after showering or to use calamine lotion, and to throw away her gardening clothes and obtain new ones.

Self-Query

Without consulting a pharmacology text, what do I know about these medications? How do these medications work?

Azithromycin

_____

_____

Prednisone

_____

_____

What is a Z-Pak, and why is it taken for only 5 days?

_____

_____

Nursing Process

What nursing assessment should be done regarding each medication? What planning and implementation do I need to do in regard to each medication? How will I evaluate each medication's effectiveness?

Azithromycin

_____

_____

Prednisone

_____

_____

Synopsis

31

Because you can find answers to the self-queries in numerous texts, you will not find the answers to all of them here. However, you will find discussion of the individual case. The scenario relates to contact dermatitis treatment; therefore, purposefully look into the medication use and vocabulary as they relate to these factors.

Vocabulary

When reviewing the vocabulary words, you might want to ask several questions: who, what, where, when, why, and how. This should give you a much broader understanding of the word.

Do yourself a favor and do not just give the shortest and simplest answer. Use the following example of vertigo: Instead of answering, "Vertigo is the feeling of the room spinning," ask:

What causes **vertigo**? Who is at risk for vertigo?

☑ Self-Query: Possible Answers

When defining the remainder of the vocabulary words, ask the following questions:

Where are **alpha cells** located? Which medications alter alpha cells?

What is an **anticholinergic effect**? How is it treated?

What are **corticosteroids**? Why are they needed?

What are **dopamine receptors**? Where are they located? Which medications alter them?

What is **folic acid**?

What is **hypochromic anemia**? How is it treated?

What is **megaloblastic anemia**? How is it treated?

What are **norepinephrine receptors**? Which medications alter them?

What are **serotonin receptors**? Which medications alter them?

What is **tyramine**? Where is it found?

What is **urushiol**? Where is it found?

(If you worked on the vocabulary words in Chapter 30, you should have most of the answers.)

Home Medications

☑ Self-Queries: Possible Answers

Aspirin (ASA) 81 mg with breakfast daily: aspirin is a salicylate that is used in numerous ways—for reducing pain, fever, and inflammation, and as an antiplatelet. In this case, it is used as an antiplatelet.

Glyburide 5 mg every 12 hours: glyburide lowers blood glucose by stimulating the pancreas to release insulin.

Hydrochlorothiazide and losartan (Hyzaar) 50/12.5, 1 tab orally daily: hydrochlorothiazide and losartan 50/12.5 is a combination medication of losartan and hydrochlorothiazide. The patient is taking it for blood pressure.

Nortriptyline (Pamelor) 20 mg at bedtime: nortriptyline belongs to the drug class called tricyclic antidepressants (TCAs) and is used to treat depression. The patient is using it as a sleeping aid.

Sertraline (Zoloft) 50 mg orally daily: sertraline is an antidepressant in a group of drugs called selective serotonin reuptake inhibitors (SSRIs). It affects chemicals in the brain.

Benadryl is an antihistamine. A side effect is drowsiness, which allows it to be used as a sleep aid as well. This individual also takes nortriptyline and sertraline. Combining the three may be additive. Diphenhydramine, because of its anticholinergic abilities, has an atropine-like action and may interact with her antihypertension medications.

Physician Orders

☑ Self-Query: Possible Answers

Azithromycin (Zithromax Z-Pak) 500 mg day 1, then 250 mg days 2–5: azithromycin is a macrolide antibiotic, used here to treat the skin infection. As you have probably discovered, there are different dosing regimens (1 day, 3 days, or 5 days). For this azithromycin, the patient takes 500 mg the first day and then 250 mg on each of the remaining 4 days.

Prednisone dose pack: prednisone is a corticosteroid. It decreases inflammation or prevents the body from responding to it. It will stop the body's response (the inflammation) to the contact with the poison ivy. Because the patient has type II diabetes mellitus, her blood glucose is expected to increase. It should return to baseline once the medication has been stopped.

Just a note: The rash is caused by the oil, called urushiol, in poison ivy. Instructing the patient to discard her old gardening clothes will help her to get rid of any lingering oil.

She was taken off the nortriptyline and remained on the sertraline. She was self-medicating and had leftover nortriptyline from a previous physician. Because the itching kept her awake at night, she decided to take the nortriptyline to sleep (she was originally prescribed the medication for this purpose). Because she had always taken the nortriptyline for sleep, she was not aware that it was also an antidepressant. This is further evidence of the need for teaching.

Case Study Inquiry

32

Vocabulary

? Self-Query

Before attempting to work the case study, define each of the vocabulary words. Although the words may have several subheadings, it will give you a place to begin your inquiry.

Dopamine receptors

_____

Folic acid

_____

Hypochromic anemia

_____

Megaloblastic anemia

_____

Norepinephrine receptors

_____

Serotonin receptors

_____

Tricyclic antidepressants

_____

Xerostomia

_____

Because you are a student, your instructor only allows you to review the patient's medications, and not the chart, to find the diagnosis. Using the medications and a pharmacology text, come up with your own idea of what the issues are for this patient.

Home Medications

Aspirin (ASA) 81 mg with breakfast daily

Calcium carbonate (Calcitrate) 250 mg with vitamin D, 1 tab orally daily

Glyburide 5 mg every 12 hours

Hydrochlorothiazide and losartan (Hyzaar) 50/12.5, 1 tab orally daily

Ibuprofen 200 mg orally daily as needed

Multivitamin for older adults orally daily

Nortriptyline (Pamelor) 20 mg at bedtime

Sertraline (Zoloft) 50 mg orally daily

Zolpidem (Ambien) 10 mg orally at bedtime

? Self-Query

Using a drug book or pharmacology text that contains the mechanism of action, unlabeled uses, and pharmacokinetics for medications, answer the following questions. Make answers specific to this scenario.

What do I know about these medications? Do I know the recommended dose of, the recommended route for, and the best time of day to give these medications? Do I know what lab results I need regarding each medication? Do I know the approved use of each medication? Do I know the most common diseases treated by the listed medications? Are any off-label uses approved for each drug?

Aspirin

_____

_____

Calcium carbonate

_____

_____

Glyburide

_____

_____

Hydrochlorothiazide and losartan

_____

_____

Ibuprofen

_____

_____

Multivitamin

_____

_____

Nortriptyline

_____

_____

Sertraline

_____

_____

Zolpidem

_____

_____

Do I know the individual's past medical history by looking at the medication list?

_____

_____

Body Systems

⁇ Self-Query

Be prepared to defend your answers.

Can I place each medication under the body system that it commonly affects?

Neurological

_____

Cardiovascular

_____

Hematological

_____

Pulmonary

_____

Gastrointestinal

_____

Nutrition

_____

Genitourinary/renal

_____

Musculoskeletal

_____

Endocrine

_____

Integumentary

_____

Immune

_____

Pain/comfort

_____

Nursing Process

⁇ Self-Query

What nursing assessment will I perform regarding each medication? What planning and implementation do I need to do in regard to each medication? How do I evaluate each medication's effectiveness?

Aspirin

_____

_____

Calcium carbonate

_____

_____

Glyburide

_____

_____

Hydrochlorothiazide and losartan

_____

_____

Ibuprofen

_____

_____

Multivitamin

_____

_____

Nortriptyline

_____

_____

Sertraline

_____

_____

Zolpidem

_____

_____

Using only the medications, complete the following:

Develop two nursing diagnoses for this patient (NANDA).

_____

_____

Develop at least three patient outcomes (NOC).

_____

_____

_____

Develop at least three patient interventions (NIC).

_____

_____

_____

Were there any duplications in the implications for the different medications? If so, explain your answer and why you think this happened.

_____

_____

_____

Synopsis

32

Because you can find answers to the self-queries in numerous texts, you will not find the answers to all of them here. However, you will find discussion of the individual case. The scenario relates to depression; therefore, purposefully look into the medication use and vocabulary as they relate to these factors.

Vocabulary

When reviewing the vocabulary words, you might want to ask several questions: who, what, where, when, why, and how. This should give you a much broader understanding of each word.

Do yourself a favor and do not just give the shortest and simplest answer. Use the following example of tricyclic antidepressants: Instead of answering, "Tricyclic antidepressants are a type of antidepressant," ask:

What are **tricyclic antidepressants**? How are they different from other antidepressants?

☑ Self-Query: Possible Answers

When defining the remainder of the vocabulary words, ask the following questions:

Where are **dopamine receptors** located? What is their function? Which medications alter them?

What is **folic acid**? What is its function?

What is **hypochromic anemia**? Why does it occur? How is it treated?

What is **megaloblastic anemia**? Why does it occur? How is it treated?

Where are **norepinephrine receptors** located? What is their function? Which medications alter them?

Where are **serotonin receptors** located? What is their function? Which medications alter them?

What is **xerostomia**? What is it caused by? How is it treated?

Home Medications

☑ Self-Query: Possible Answers

Aspirin (ASA) 81 mg with breakfast daily: aspirin is a salicylate that is used in numerous ways—for reducing pain, fever, and inflammation, and as an antiplatelet. In this case, it is used as an antiplatelet.

Calcium carbonate (Calcitrate) 250 mg with vitamin D, 1 tab orally daily: calcium and vitamin D supplement.

Glyburide 5 mg every 12 hours: medication lowers blood glucose by stimulating the pancreas to release insulin.

Hydrochlorothiazide and losartan (Hyzaar) 50/12.5, 1 tab orally daily: hydrochlorothiazide and losartan 50/12.5 is a combination medication of losartan and hydrochlorothiazide. The patient is taking it for blood pressure.

Ibuprofen 200 mg orally daily as needed: ibuprofen is a nonsteroidal anti-inflammatory drug (NSAID) used for pain relief in this individual.

Multivitamin for older adults orally daily: nutrient supplement intake.

Nortriptyline (Pamelor) 20 mg at bedtime: nortriptyline belongs to the drug class called tricyclic anti-depressants (TCAs) and is used for treating depression. The patient began using it many years ago and uses it as a sleeping aid.

Sertraline (Zoloft) 50 mg orally daily: sertraline is a selective serotonin reuptake inhibitor (SSRI) and acts as an antidepressant.

Zolpidem (Ambien) 10 mg orally at bedtime: zolpidem is a sedative/hypnotic approved for the short-term treatment of insomnia. It usually works within 30 minutes.

Body Systems

☑ Self-Query: Possible Answers

Neurological

> Sertraline
> Zolpidem
> Aventyl

Cardiovascular

> Hydrochlorothiazide and losartan
> Aspirin

Hematological

> Aspirin

Pulmonary

> None specific

Gastrointestinal

> Calcium carbonate 250 mg with vitamin D (What is vitamin D's effect on calcium in the small intestine?)

Nutrition

> Micronase
> Multivitamin for older adults

Genitourinary/renal

> Hydrochlorothiazide and losartan (See the medication combination in this drug.)

Musculoskeletal

> Ibuprofen

Endocrine

> Micronase alters the production of insulin in the pancreas.

Integumentary

> None specific

Immune

    None specific

Pain/comfort

    Ibuprofen

Nursing Process

☑ Self-Query: Possible Answers

Discussion with the class about duplications in the implications for different medications should center on:

    Aventyl 20 mg
    Sertraline 50 mg
    Zolpidem 10 mg

Case Study Inquiry

33

Vocabulary

Self-Query

Before attempting to work the case study, define each of the vocabulary words. Although the words may have several subheadings, it will give you a place to begin your inquiry.

Benzodiazepine
_____

Bezoar formation
_____

Folic acid
_____

Gastric ulcers
_____

Hypochromic anemia
_____

Intrinsic factor
_____

Serotonin receptors
_____

Xerostomia
_____

Because you are a student, your instructor only allows you to review the patient's medications, and not the chart, to find the diagnosis. Using the medications and a pharmacology text, come up with your own idea of what the issues are for this patient.

Home Medications

Ferrous sulfate 300 mg twice daily with meals
Lorazepam (Ativan) 1 mg orally, 1–2 every 2–4 hours as needed
Sucralfate 1 g twice a day 1 hour before meals
Thiamine hydrochloride (B1) 100-mg tab daily
Venlafaxine (Effexor) XR 75 mg orally daily
Vitamin B12 200 mcg intramuscularly monthly

Self-Query

Using a drug book or pharmacology text that contains the mechanism of action, unlabeled uses, and pharmacokinetics for medications, answer the following questions. Make answers specific to this scenario.

What do I know about these medications? Do I know the recommended dose of, the recommended route for, and the best time of day to give these medications? Do I know what lab results I need regarding each medication? Do I know the approved use of each medication? Do I know the most common diseases treated by the listed medications? Are any off-label uses approved for each drug?

Ferrous sulfate

_____

_____

Lorazepam

_____

_____

Sucralfate

_____

_____

Thiamine hydrochloride

_____

_____

Venlafaxine

_____

_____

Vitamin B12

_____

_____

Do I know the individual's past medical history by looking at the medication list?

_____

_____

Body Systems

Self-Query

Be prepared to defend your answers.

Can I place each medication under the body system that it commonly affects?

Neurological

_____

Cardiovascular

_____

Hematological

_____

Pulmonary

_____

Gastrointestinal

_____

Nutrition

_____

Genitourinary/renal

_____

Musculoskeletal

_____

Endocrine

_____

Integumentary

_____

Immune

_____

Pain/comfort

_____

Nursing Process

Self-Query

What nursing assessment will I perform regarding each medication? What planning and implementation do I need to do in regard to each medication? How do I evaluate each medication's effectiveness?

Ferrous sulfate

_____

_____

Lorazepam

_____

_____

Sucralfate

_____

_____

Thiamine hydrochloride

_____

_____

Venlafaxine

_____

_____

Vitamin B12

_____

_____

Using only the medications, complete the following:

Develop two nursing diagnoses for this patient (NANDA).

_____

_____

Develop at least three patient outcomes (NOC).

_____

_____

Develop at least three patient interventions (NIC).

_____

_____

Synopsis

33

Because you can find answers to the self-queries in numerous texts, you will not find the answers to all of them here. However, you will find discussion of the individual case. The scenario relates to anemia. Therefore, purposefully look into the medication use and vocabulary as they relate to these factors.

Vocabulary

When reviewing the vocabulary words, you might want to ask several questions: who, what, where, when, why, and how. This should give you a much broader understanding of each word.

Do yourself a favor and do not just give the shortest and simplest answer. Use the following example of benzodiazepine: Instead of answering, "Benzodiazepines are drugs that alter the central nervous system," ask:

Who is prescribed a **benzodiazepine**? Are the effects dose related?

☑ Self-Query: Possible Answers

When defining the remainder of the vocabulary words, ask the following questions:

What causes a **bezoar** formation? How is it treated?

What is **folic acid**? Why is it needed in the body?

Who develops **gastric ulcers**? What are the medications prescribed for gastric ulcers?

What is **hypochromic anemia**? What medications can cause it? What medications can treat it?

What is the **intrinsic factor**? Where is it located? Why is it needed?

What are **serotonin receptors**? What medications affect them?

What is **xerostomia**? What medications can cause it?

Home Medications

☑ Self-Query: Possible Answers

Ferrous sulfate 300 mg twice daily with meals: an essential trace mineral vital to human nutrition, iron is crucial to the entire process of respiration, including electron and oxygen transport. Iron is essential to the production and performance of hemoglobin, which carries nearly all the oxygen in the blood to needed locations throughout the body. Too little iron in the body's system can lead to microcytic hypochromic anemia.

Sucralfate 1 g twice a day 1 hour before meals: sucralfate works mainly by coating an ulcer located in the lining of the stomach. It protects the area from digestive materials used by the body for digestion of food. Sucralfate treats an active duodenal ulcer; it can heal an active ulcer, but it will not prevent future ulcers from occurring. Prevention should be discussed.

Thiamine hydrochloride (B1) 100-mg tab daily: vitamin B1 is water soluble and is used by the body to help process protein, fat, and carbohydrates. The vitamin is also used by nerve cells to help them function correctly.

Venlafaxine (Effexor) XR 75 mg orally daily: venlafaxine is used for depression and generalized anxiety. Note that this is a selective serotonin and norepinephrine reuptake inhibitor (SSNRI), not just a selective serotonin reuptake inhibitor (SSRI).

Vitamin B12 200 mcg intramuscularly monthly: intake of vitamin B12 is critical for bodily functions. It works with folate to create building blocks for RNA and DNA synthesis. Vitamin B12 works in the nervous system. It works with vitamin B6 and folic acid to control levels of homocysteine.

☑ Self-Query: Possible Answers

At first glance, the individual has a history of depression (maybe). There are off-label uses for this medication:

Pernicious anemia
Active ulcer

Body Systems

☑ Self-Query: Possible Answers

Neurological

Venlafaxine XR 75 mg orally daily

Cardiovascular

None noted

Hematological

None noted

Pulmonary

None noted

Gastrointestinal

Sucralfate 1 g
Vitamin B12 200 mcg
Ferrous sulfate 300 mg (consider constipation issues)

Nutrition

Vitamin B12 200 mcg
Ferrous sulfate 300 mg
Sucralfate 1 g (not given within an hour of meals; it decreases absorption by coating the lining of the stomach)
Thiamine hydrochloride 100 mg

Genitourinary/renal

None specific

Musculoskeletal

None specific

Endocrine

None specific

Integumentary

    None specific

Immune

    None specific

Pain/comfort

    Venlafaxine XR 75 mg orally daily

Nursing Process

☑ Self-Query: Possible Answers

Upon assessment and reviewing labs, you may realize that the individual has pernicious anemia. The ulcer that has been treated in the past and that improved with sucralfate was not responding to this treatment, and the individual needed a further workup for possible *Helicobacter pylori*. After a thorough assessment and medication history, it was revealed that the individual was also taking an antacid with the sucralfate thinking that it would be beneficial. Unfortunately, sucralfate needs an acid medium to work, and the antacid was negating the therapeutic effect. After education, therapy was restarted, and this time, the ulcer was treated effectively.

Case Study Inquiry

34

Vocabulary

? **Self-Query**

Before attempting to work the case study, define each of the vocabulary words. Although the words may have several subheadings, it will give you a place to begin your inquiry.

Cellulitis

_____

High-density lipoprotein (HDL)

_____

Hypothyroidism

_____

Low-density lipoprotein (LDL)

_____

Nicotine

_____

Nicotine receptors

_____

Prostaglandin

_____

Triglycerides

_____

A 55-year-old female is in the office today for follow-up on a leg wound. Her leg was red and filled with blood and pus. She scraped it on a woodpile while carrying wood to her fireplace. Using the medications and a pharmacology text, come up with your own idea of what the issues are for this patient.

Home Medications

Acetaminophen/propoxyphene (Darvocet-N 100) 1–2 orally every 8 hours as needed

Bupropion 150 mg orally every 8 hours

Cephalexin (Keflex) 500 mg orally every 8 hours

Fluticasone propionate/salmeterol (Advair Diskus) 500/50, 1 dose every 12 hours

Levothyroxine (Synthroid) 0.125 mg orally

Methylprednisolone (Solu-Medrol) 125 mg IV every 8 hours

Normal saline IV at 30 mL/hr (KVO)

Regular insulin sliding scale with Accu-checks 7-11-4-9

Theophylline (Theo-Dur) 300 mg orally every 12 hours

Self-Query

Using a drug book or pharmacology text that contains the mechanism of action, unlabeled uses, and pharmacokinetics for medications, answer the following questions. Make answers specific to this scenario.

What do I know about these medications? Do I know the recommended dose of, the recommended route for, and the best time of day to give these medications? Do I know what lab results I need regarding each medication? Do I know the approved use of each medication? Do I know the most common diseases treated by the listed medications? Are any off-label uses approved for each drug?

Acetaminophen/propoxyphene

_____

_____

Bupropion

_____

_____

Cephalexin

_____

_____

Fluticasone propionate/salmeterol

_____

_____

Levothyroxine

_____

_____

Methylprednisolone

_____

_____

Normal saline

_____

_____

Regular insulin

_____

_____

Theophylline

_____

_____

What does "sliding scale" indicate?

_____

Do the fluticasone propionate/salmeterol and methylprednisolone affect the way the patient responds to infections? (Explain your answer.)

_____

_____

Why assess the oral status for candida on this patient?

_____

What are two uses for bupropion?

_____

Do I know the individual's past medical history by looking at the medication list?

_____

_____

Body Systems

❓ Self-Query

Be prepared to defend your answers.

Can I place each medication under the body system that it commonly affects?

Neurological

_____

Cardiovascular

_____

Hematological

_____

Pulmonary

_____

Gastrointestinal

_____

Nutrition

_____

Genitourinary/renal

_____

Musculoskeletal

_____

Endocrine

_____

Integumentary

_____

Immune

_____

Pain/comfort

_____

Nursing Process

❓ Self-Query

What nursing assessment will I perform for each medication? What planning and implementation do I need to do in regard to each medication? How do I evaluate each medication's effectiveness?

Acetaminophen/propoxyphene

_____

_____

Bupropion

_____

_____

Cephalexin

_____

_____

Fluticasone propionate/salmeterol

_____

_____

Levothyroxine

_____

_____

Methylprednisolone

_____

_____

Normal saline

_____

_____

Regular insulin

_____

_____

Theophylline

_____

_____

Physician Orders

Daptomycin (Cubicin)

You are to contact a home infusion company of the patient's choice and begin IV daptomycin. The pharmacist at the infusion company will collaborate with the physician. This is a new medication, so you look it up to educate the patient (and yourself).

Calculated by body weight

Relatively new IV mediation

Once-daily 30-minute low-volume infusion

Does not require drug levels to be drawn

Low potential for drug–drug interactions

Using only the medications, complete the following for each medication:

⁂ Self-Query

Develop two nursing diagnoses for this patient (NANDA).

_____

_____

Develop at least three patient outcomes (NOC).

_____

_____

_____

Develop at least three patient interventions (NIC).

_____

_____

_____

Synopsis

34

Because you can find answers to the self-queries in numerous texts, you will not find the answers to all of them here. However, you will find discussion of the individual case. The scenario relates to medication-induced immunodeficiency; therefore, purposefully look into medication use and vocabulary as they relate to these factors.

Vocabulary

When reviewing the vocabulary words, you might want to ask several questions: who, what, where, when, why, and how. This should give you a much broader understanding of each word.

Do yourself a favor and do not just give the shortest and simplest answer. Use the following example of cellulitis: Instead of answering, "Cellulitis is inflammation of the tissue," ask:

What causes **cellulitis**? Who is at risk for cellulitis?

☑ Self-Query: Possible Answers

When defining the vocabulary words, ask the following questions:

Where is **high-density lipoprotein (HDL)** stored in the body?

How does **hypothyroidism** affect the cardiac system? In what system does it belong? What lab values are monitored?

How is **low-density lipoprotein (LDL)** different from HDL?

What affect does **nicotine** have on the endocrine and cardiac systems?

How are **nicotinic receptors** activated? What response is seem in the body when they are activated?

Where does the term **prostaglandins** originate? How are prostaglandins beneficial? How are they detrimental?

How are **triglycerides** beneficial? How are they detrimental? How are these monitored?

Home Medications

☑ Self-Query: Possible Answers

Acetaminophen/propoxyphene (Darvocet-N 100) 1-2 orally every 8 hours as needed: acetaminophen/propoxyphene is a combination analgesic. Each tablet contains 100 mg propoxyphene and 650 mg of acetaminophen. Propoxyphene is considered an opioid pain reliever. Acetaminophen is a nonopioid pain reliever. The combination of acetaminophen and propoxyphene enhances the effect of each medication.

Bupropion 150 mg orally every 8 hours: bupropion (Wellbutrin) is an atypical antidepressant that acts on norepinephrine, dopamine, and nicotinic receptors. The patient takes bupropion because the disease creates a great deal of anxiety. The aminophylline dose creates anxiety and jitters. Bupropion, marketed as Zyban, also has been found to be an effective smoking cessation aid.

Cephalexin (Keflex) 500 mg every 8 hours orally: cephalexin is from a previous office visit for infection. This is to be stopped. Because of her lung disease, the patient is on corticosteroids, which decreases her immunity and thus her body's ability to fight off an infection.

Fluticasone propionate/salmeterol (Advair Diskus) 500/50, 1 dose every 12 hours: fluticasone propionate/salmeterol contains salmeterol, a beta-2 agonist bronchodilator, and fluticasone, an anti-inflammatory corticosteroid.

Levothyroxine (Synthroid) 0.125 mg orally: levothyroxine is a thyroid hormone replacement.

Theophylline (Theo-Dur) 300 mg orally every 12 hours: theophylline contains the medicine aminophylline/theophylline and belongs to the group of medicines called xanthine, which act as bronchodilators. Another xanthine derivative, caffeine, can be used as a stimulant. Levels must be drawn on this medication.

Prednisone 5 mg orally daily: prednisone is a synthetic corticosteroid effective as an immuno-suppressant.

Insulin glargine (Lantus) 30 units subcutaneously at bedtime: 24-hour *insulin* approved exclusively for use once a day. The patient is a type II diabetic. Take note of all her medications, particularly the steroids.

Because of her lung disease, the patient is on corticosteroids, which decreases her immunity and thus decreases her body's ability to fight off an infection. She and her primary care provider took great care in determining the amount of prednisone she needs to reduce the inflammation in her lungs. Dosing of long-term corticosteroid involves several stages:

(1) The initial dose is given to control the inflammation.
(2) The dose is decreased to a maintenance dose that continues to suppress inflammation.
(3) Continuing the maintenance dose until tapering off corticosteroids is established.
(4) The decision is made to decrease the dose and withdraw the steroids.
(5) During the decrease in dose, her symptoms return.
(6) She is maintained at 5 mg prednisone.

You should assess the oral status for candida on this patient because antibiotics and steroids are major factors in the growth of candida.

Body Systems

☑ Self-Queries: Possible Answers

Neurological

Bupropion 150 mg

Theophylline may cause CNS stimulation (similar to caffeine, another xanthine). Therapeutic levels must be maintained between 5 and 15 mcg/mL.

Cardiovascular

None specific. However, theophylline may cause cardiac stimulation.

Hematological

Cephalexin 500 mg
Prednisone 5 mg

Pulmonary

Prednisone 5 mg
Fluticasone propionate/salmeterol 500/50
Theophylline 300 mg

Gastrointestinal

None specific. However, prednisone 5 mg will cause GI upset.

Nutrition

None specific. However, corticosteroids cause glucose metabolism issues.

Genitourinary/renal

None specific

Musculoskeletal

None specific. However, corticosteroids increase the risk for osteoporosis.

Endocrine

Prednisone 5 mg (synthetic corticosteroid)
Insulin glargine 30 units
Levothyroxine 0.125 (has thyroid levels drawn regularly)

Integumentary

Cephalexin 500 mg (under the system infected)

Immune

Prednisone 5 mg (actually alters every aspect of the immune system)

Pain/comfort

Acetaminophen/propoxyphene

Nursing Process

☑ Self-Query: Possible Answers

The goal is to treat the infection and keep the patient on her present medications. Cubicin is being ordered when not cost prohibited.

Case Study Inquiry

35

Vocabulary

Self-Query

Before attempting to work the case study, define each of the vocabulary words. Although the words may have several subheadings, it will give you a place to begin your inquiry.

Cholesterol
_____

Grave's disease
_____

Hypothyroidism
_____

Low-density lipoprotein (LDL)
_____

Nicotine receptors
_____

Prostaglandin
_____

Substance abuse
_____

Transdermal medication
_____

Triglycerides
_____

A 68-year-old male is in the office today seeking help in stopping smoking. Using the medications and a pharmacology text, come up with your own idea of what the issues are for this patient.

Home Medications

Acetaminophen/propoxyphene (Darvocet-N 100) 1–2 orally every 8 hours as needed

Aspirin (ASA) 81 mg orally daily

Fluticasone propionate/salmeterol (Advair Diskus) 500/50, 1 dose every 12 hours

Gemfibrozil 600 mg orally 1 tab before breakfast

Levothyroxine (Synthroid) 0.125 mg orally

Spironolactone 25 mg 1 tab orally daily

? Self-Query

Using a drug book or pharmacology text that contains the mechanism of action, unlabeled uses, and pharmacokinetics for medications, answer the following questions. Make answers specific to this scenario.

What do I know about these medications? Do I know the recommended dose of, the recommended route for, and the best time of day to give these medications? Do I know what lab results I need regarding each medication? Do I know the approved use of each medication? Do I know the most common diseases treated by the listed medications? Are any off-label uses approved for each drug?

Acetaminophen/propoxyphene

_____

_____

Aspirin

_____

_____

Fluticasone propionate/salmeterol

_____

_____

Gemfibrozil

_____

_____

Levothyroxine

_____

_____

Spironolactone

_____

_____

Does the fluticasone propionate/salmeterol affect the way the patient responds to infections? (Explain your answer.)

_____

_____

What are two uses for bupropion?

_____

Do I know the individual's past medical history by looking at the medication list?

_____

_____

Body Systems

🔖 Self-Query

Be prepared to defend your answers.

Can I place each medication under the body system that it commonly affects?

Neurological

_____

Cardiovascular

_____

Hematological

_____

Pulmonary

_____

Gastrointestinal

_____

Nutrition

_____

Genitourinary/renal

_____

Musculoskeletal

_____

Endocrine

_____

Integumentary

_____

Immune

_____

Pain/comfort

_____

Nursing Process

🔖 Self-Query

What nursing assessment will I perform for each medication? What planning and implementation do I need to do in regard to each medication? How do I evaluate each medication's effectiveness?

Acetaminophen/propoxyphene

_____

_____

Aspirin

_____

_____

Fluticasone propionate/salmeterol

_____

_____

Gemfibrozil

_____

_____

Levothyroxine

_____

_____

Spironolactone

_____

_____

Using only the medications, complete the following for each medication:

Develop two nursing diagnoses for this patient (NANDA).

_____

_____

Develop at least three patient outcomes (NOC).

_____

_____

_____

Develop at least three patient interventions (NIC).

_____

_____

_____

Physician Orders

The physician has placed the man on a nicotine patch, 14 mg to begin. He is to return to the office in 2 weeks for assessment and a different dose.

? Self-Query

Write a teaching plan for this patient regarding the nicotine and the way the patch will work.

_____

_____

_____

<h1>Synopsis</h1>

<h1>35</h1>

Because you can find answers to the self-queries in numerous texts, you will not find the answers to all of them here. However, you will find discussion of the individual case. The scenario relates to pulmonary disease and smoking cessation; therefore, purposefully look into the medication use and vocabulary as they relate to these factors.

Vocabulary

When reviewing the vocabulary words, you might want to ask several questions: who, what, where, when, why, and how. This should give you a much broader understanding of each word.

Do yourself a favor and do not just give the shortest and simplest answer. Use the following example of cholesterol: Instead of answering, "Cholesterol is a lipid found in the body," ask:

Why do we have **cholesterol**? Where do we obtain cholesterol? What is the classification of medications that treat high cholesterol?

☑ Self-Query: Possible Answers

When defining the remainder of the vocabulary words, ask the following questions:

What is **Grave's disease**? Which medications treat Grave's disease? Who is at risk for Grave's disease?

What are **nicotine receptors**? Where are they located? Are they connected to nicotine addiction?

How do **transdermal medications** work? How are they absorbed? Which medications can be given transdermally?

What are **triglycerides**? How do the levels of a person's triglycerides affect his or her medications?

How is **substance abuse** defined? Who is at risk for addiction? Are all medications capable of being abused?

How does the **low-density lipoprotein (LDL)** level affect medication administration?

Home Medications

☑ Self-Query: Possible Answers

Acetaminophen/propoxyphene (Darvocet-N 100) 1–2 orally every 8 hours as needed: acetaminophen/propoxyphene is a combination analgesic. Each tablet contains 100 mg propoxyphene and 650 mg acetaminophen. Propoxyphene is considered an opioid pain reliever, and acetaminophen is a nonopioid pain reliever. The combination of acetaminophen and propoxyphene enhances the effect of each medication.

Aspirin (ASA) 81 mg orally daily: aspirin is a salicylate that is used in numerous ways—for pain, fever, and inflammation reduction, and as an antiplatelet. In this case, it is used as an antiplatelet medication.

Fluticasone propionate/salmeterol (Advair Diskus) 500/50, 1 dose every 12 hours: fluticasone propionate/salmeterol contains salmeterol, a beta-2 agonist bronchodilator, and fluticasone, an anti-inflammatory corticosteroid. Long-term use of corticosteroids can increase the risk of osteoporosis and decrease the body's ability to fight infections.

Gemfibrozil 600 mg orally 1 tab before breakfast: gemfibrozil is a lipid-regulating agent. It raises HDL and decreases triglycerides. It is classified as a fibric acid derivative. Gemfibrozil is prescribed after other therapies have failed, and it is not intended for treating patients who only have low HDL. The patient's triglycerides were high enough to cause damage to his pancreas if not treated.

Spironolactone 25 mg 1 tab orally daily: potassium-sparing diuretic; it increases the excretion of water and sodium.

Body Systems

☑ Self-Queries: Possible Answers

Neurological

> Acetaminophen/propoxyphene 1–2 orally every 8 as needed

Cardiovascular

> Spironolactone 25 mg—affects cardiovascular system through fluid regulation
> Gemfibrozil 600 mg
> Aspirin 81 mg—has many functions; used as an antiplatelet in this case

Hematological

> Gemfibrozil 600—alters HDL and LDL
> Aspirin 81 mg—interferes with platelet aggregation

Pulmonary

> Fluticasone propionate/salmeterol 500/50, 1 dose every 12 hours

Gastrointestinal

> Aspirin 81 mg—not a GI medication, but be aware of the alterations to the lining of the GI tract due to the decrease in prostaglandin production.

Nutrition

> None specific

Genitourinary/renal

> Spironolactone 25 mg—potassium-sparing diuretic
> Aspirin 81 mg—not a renal medication, but be aware of the alterations to renal perfusion due to the decrease in prostaglandin production.

Musculoskeletal

> Acetaminophen/propoxyphene 1–2 orally every 8 hours as needed

Endocrine

> None specific

Integumentary

> None specific

Immune

Fluticasone propionate/salmeterol 500/50

Pain/comfort

Acetaminophen/propoxyphene 1–2 orally every 8 hours as needed
Aspirin 81 mg
Nicotine patch 14 mg

Nursing Process

☑ Self-Query: Possible Answers

A nicotine patch is a transdermal medication that releases nicotine into the body through the skin. Nicotine patches typically come in three different dosage strengths: 21 mg, 14 mg, and 7 mg; the number refers to the amount of nicotine in the patch. This man will begin at the higher end because he smokes 20 cigarettes a day. Depending on his progress, he will be prescribed a lower dose when he returns. These patches are available over the counter. However, he has cardiac risk factors and wanted to be placed under a physician's care. The teaching plan should be group discussion.

Case Study Inquiry

36

Vocabulary

? Self-Query

Before attempting to work the case study, define each of the vocabulary words. Although the words may have several subheadings, it will give you a place to begin your inquiry.

Addison's disease

_____

Carbohydrates

_____

Cushing's disease

_____

Glucose tolerance test

_____

HgbA1C

_____

Parathyroid

_____

Proteins

_____

Thyroid

_____

A 68-year-old male in the office today states that his blood sugar machine is not working because every morning his blood sugar reads 200, and he wants to know why. Using the medications and a pharmacology text, come up with your own idea of what the issues are for this patient.

Home Medications

Carvedilol (Coreg) 6.25 mg every 12 hours

Clopidogrel (Plavix) 75 mg orally daily

Fenofibrate (TriCor) 48-mg tab orally daily

Irbesartan (Avapro) 150 mg orally every 12 hours

Pioglitazone (Actos) 15 mg orally daily

Psyllium (Metamucil) 1 dose as instructed on bottle every morning with breakfast

Vitamin E 400-unit capsule orally daily

Using a drug book or pharmacology text that contains the mechanism of action, unlabeled uses, and pharmacokinetics of medications, answer the following questions. Make answers specific to this scenario.

What do I know about these medications? Do I know the recommended dose of, the recommended route for, and the best time of day to give these medications? Do I know what lab results I need regarding each medication? Do I know the approved use of each medication? Do I know the most common diseases treated by the listed medications? Are any off-label uses approved for each drug?

Carvedilol

_____

_____

Clopidogrel

_____

_____

Fenofibrate

_____

_____

Irbesartan

_____

_____

Pioglitazone

_____

_____

Psyllium

_____

_____

Vitamin E

_____

_____

Physician Orders

After lab results report that the FBS is elevated (and it is not the patient's glucometer), the physician prescribes:

Metformin (Glucophage) 500 mg orally daily to be taken with his other antidiabetic drug

☞ **Self-Query**

Match the patient's medications to his medical history. The patient has a medical history of:

Coronary artery disease (CAD)

_____

Hypertension

_____

Diabetes mellitus type II

Diverticulitis

Body Systems

Self-Query

Be prepared to defend your answers.

Can I place each medication under the body system that it commonly affects?

Neurological

Cardiovascular

Hematological

Pulmonary

Gastrointestinal

Nutrition

Genitourinary/renal

Musculoskeletal

Endocrine

Integumentary

Immune

Pain/comfort

Nursing Process

Self-Query

What nursing assessment will I perform for each medication? What planning and implementation do I need to do in regard to each medication? How do I evaluate each medication's effectiveness?

Carvedilol

Clopidogrel

_____

_____

Fenofibrate

_____

_____

Irbesartan

_____

_____

Pioglitazone

_____

_____

Psyllium

_____

_____

Vitamin E

_____

_____

Using only the medications, complete the following for each medication:

Develop two nursing diagnoses for this patient (NANDA).

_____

_____

Develop at least three patient outcomes (NOC).

_____

_____

Develop at least three patient interventions (NIC).

_____

_____

_____

Synopsis

36

Because you can find answers to the self-queries in numerous texts, you will not find the answers to all of them here. However, you will find discussion of the individual case. The scenario relates to cardiac and diabetes issues; therefore, purposefully look into the medication use and vocabulary as they relate to these factors.

Vocabulary

When reviewing the vocabulary words, you might want to ask several questions: who, what, where, when, why, and how. This should give you a much broader understanding of each word.

Do yourself a favor and do not just give the shortest and simplest answer. Use the following example of the glucose tolerance test: Instead of answering, "A glucose tolerance test is a test to check for diabetes," ask:

Why is the **glucose tolerance test** done? Who needs to have the test completed?

☑ Self-Query: Possible Answers

When defining the remainder of the vocabulary words, ask the following questions:

What is **Addison's disease**? Who is at risk? What medications can cause it? What medications can treat it?

What are **carbohydrates**? Where are they found?

What is **Cushing's disease**? Who is at risk for Cushing's? What medications can cause it? What medications can treat it?

What is the **HgbA1C**? Who has it tested? What does it reveal?

What is the function of the **parathyroid**? How can its functioning be disrupted?

What are **proteins**? Where are they found? What is their function in the body in relation to medications?

What is the function of the **thyroid**? How can its functioning be disrupted?

Home Medications

☑ Self-Query: Possible Answers

Carvedilol (Coreg) 6.25 mg every 12 hours: carvedilol is an alpha-1 beta blocker used to treat hypertension. Note that this individual has diabetes. He was prescribed pioglitazone (Actos), and now metformin. The medications together can potentiate hypoglycemia. Carvedilol can mask early warning symptoms of hypoglycemia such as tachycardia. Tachycardia in hypoglycemia is due to activation of the adrenergic nervous system. Carvedilol, being a beta blocker, blocks this reaction. This is an education issue; all diabetics should be made aware of this when they start a beta blocker.

Clopidogrel (Plavix) 75 mg orally daily: clopidogrel is an anticoagulant (that is, it keeps platelets from sticking together). It is used to prevent myocardial infarctions and cerebral vascular accidents.

Fenofibrate (TriCor) 48-mg tab orally daily: fenofibrate is used as a lipid-lowering agent. It promotes the control of elevated cholesterol and triglyceride levels in the blood. This is the lowest dose of the medication. After 6 weeks on the medication, the healthcare provider will monitor blood work to see if the cholesterol and triglyceride levels are decreasing. If so, the patient will remain at this dose; if not, his dose will be increased.

Irbesartan (Avapro) 150 mg orally every 12 hours: irbesartan is an angiotensin II receptor antagonist used to treat hypertension.

Pioglitazone 15 mg orally daily: pioglitazone stimulates the cells so that the cell is more sensitive to insulin.

Psyllium (Metamucil) 1 dose as instructed on bottle every morning with breakfast: psyllium is a bulk-forming laxative that the patient used for diverticulitis. It increases liquid in the stool, making it softer and easier to pass. This may not be the best medication for this geriatric individual because his fluid intake may not be adequate.

Vitamin E 400-unit capsule orally daily: vitamin E is a fat-soluble vitamin used as an antioxidant. The healthcare provider needs to monitor for bleeding tendencies in a patient who is also taking clopidogrel.

Physician Orders

Metformin (Glucophage) 500 mg orally daily to be taken with his other antidiabetic drug: metformin stimulates the cells so that they are more sensitive to insulin, decreases liver production of glucose, and decreases the uptake of glucose in the intestines.

☑ Self-Query: Possible Answers

The patient's medications match up with his medical history as follows:

CAD

> Irbesartan 150 mg orally every 12 hours
> Carvedilol 6.25 mg every 12 hours
> Clopidogrel 75 mg orally daily
> Vitamin E 400-unit capsule orally daily
> Fenofibrate 48-mg tab orally daily

Hypertension

> Irbesartan 150 mg orally every 12 hours
> Carvedilol 6.25 mg every 12 hours

Diabetes mellitus type II

> Pioglitazone 15 mg orally daily

Diverticulitis

> Psyllium 1 dose as instructed on bottle every morning with breakfast
> Pioglitazone 15 mg orally daily
> Irbesartan 150 mg orally every 12 hours
> Carvedilol 6.25 mg every 12 hours
> Clopidogrel 75 mg orally daily
> Vitamin E 400-unit capsule orally daily
> Fenofibrate 48-mg tab orally daily
> Metformin 500 mg orally daily

Body Systems

Neurological

None specific

Cardiovascular

Irbesartan 150 mg orally every 12 hours
Carvedilol 6.25 mg every 12 hours
Clopidogrel 75 mg orally daily
Vitamin E 400-unit capsule orally daily
Fenofibrate 48-mg tab orally daily

Hematological

Clopidogrel 75 mg orally daily
Vitamin E 400-unit capsule orally daily
Fenofibrate 48-mg tab orally daily

Pulmonary

None specific

Gastrointestinal

None specific; however, metformin and pioglitazone function in the gastrointestinal tract.
Psyllium 1 dose as instructed on bottle every morning with breakfast
Metformin 500 mg orally daily to be taken with patient's other antidiabetic drug

Nutrition

Metformin and pioglitazone function at the cellular level to increase the use of glucose. Metformin stimulates the cells so that they are more sensitive to insulin, decreases liver production of glucose, and decreases the uptake of glucose in the intestines.

Genitourinary/renal

Irbesartan 150 mg orally every 12 hours

Musculoskeletal

None specific; however, pioglitazone and metformin function at the cellular level to increase the use of glucose in muscle cells.

Endocrine

None specific. Some students may place metformin and pioglitazone here. They need to give a rationale given that these medications do not alter the endocrine organs.

Integumentary

None specific

Immune

None specific

Pain/comfort

None specific

Nursing Process

☑ Self-Query: Possible Answers

Group discussion should center on the connection of diabetes to hypertension and cardiac disease.

Case Study Inquiry

37

Vocabulary

Self-Query

Before attempting to work the case study, define each of the vocabulary words. Although the words may have several subheadings, it will give you a place to begin your inquiry.

Anxiety

_____

Asthma

_____

Gout

_____

Hyperlipidemia

_____

Hypertension

_____

Hypothyroidism

_____

Left heart failure

_____

This case involves follow-up care related to hypovolemic acute renal failure in a 68-year-old male. The patient is at risk for falls because of an inability to maintain balance. He lives in a split-level home in which the kitchen and bedroom are on different levels.

Home Medications

Acetaminophen and hydrocodone (Anexsia) 7.5/650 orally 1–2 tabs every 4 hours as needed

Albuterol (90 mcg) 2 puffs every 4 hours as needed

Allopurinol 300 mg orally daily

Bumetanide (Bumex) 1 mg orally daily

Buspirone 30 mg orally every 12 hours

Digoxin 0.125 mg orally daily

Docusate/sennoside (Senokot-S) 2 pills daily as needed

Levothyroxine 0.1 mg orally daily

Lisinopril 10 mg orally daily

Mometasone 220 mcg daily inhalation

Nebivolol 5 mg orally daily

Omeprazole (Prilosec) 40 mg daily orally

Warfarin 2 mg orally daily

? Self-Query

Using a drug book or pharmacology text that contains the mechanism of action, unlabeled uses, and pharmacokinetics of medications, answer the following questions. Make answers specific to this scenario.

What do I know about these medications? Do I know the recommended dose of, the recommended route for, and the best time of day to give these medications? Do I know what lab results I need regarding each medication? Do I know the approved use of each medication? Do I know the most common diseases treated by the listed medications? Are any off-label uses approved for each drug?

Acetaminophen and hydrocodone

_____

_____

Albuterol

_____

_____

Allopurinol

_____

_____

Bumetanide

_____

_____

Buspirone

_____

_____

Digoxin

_____

_____

Docusate/sennoside

_____

_____

Levothyroxine

_____

_____

Lisinopril

_____

_____

Mometasone

_____

_____

Nebivolol

_____

_____

Omeprazole

_____

_____

Warfarin

_____

_____

How do these medications interact with each other?

_____

_____

Reviewing the medications, what is the patient's possible past medical history?

_____

_____

Nursing Process

Self-Query

What nursing assessment should be performed for each medication? What planning and implementation are needed in regard to each medication? How do I evaluate each medication's effectiveness?

Acetaminophen and hydrocodone

_____

_____

Albuterol

_____

_____

Allopurinol

_____

_____

Bumetanide

_____

_____

Buspirone

_____

_____

Digoxin

_____

_____

Docusate/sennoside

_____

_____

Levothyroxine

_____

_____

Lisinopril

_____

_____

Mometasone

_____

_____

Nebivolol

_____

_____

Omeprazole

_____

_____

Warfarin

_____

_____

_____

Body Systems

🔍 Self-Query

Be prepared to defend your answers.

Can I place each medication under the body system that it commonly affects?

Neurological

_____

Cardiovascular

_____

Hematological

_____

Pulmonary

_____

Gastrointestinal

_____

Nutrition

_____

Genitourinary/renal

_____

Musculoskeletal

_____

Endocrine

_____

Integumentary

_____

Immune

_____

Pain/comfort

_____

Nursing Process

Self-Query

Develop two nursing diagnoses for this patient (NANDA).

_____

_____

Develop at least three patient outcomes (NOC).

_____

_____

_____

Develop at least three patient interventions (NIC).

_____

_____

_____

What do you think may have caused the dehydration that led to the acute renal failure?

_____

_____

Synopsis

37

Because you can find answers to the self-queries in numerous texts, you will not find the answers to all of them here. However, you will find discussion of the individual cases. The scenario relates to medication-induced immunodeficiency; therefore, purposefully look into the medication use and vocabulary as they relate to these factors.

Vocabulary

When reviewing the vocabulary words, you might want to ask several questions: who, what, where, when, why, and how. This should give you a much broader understanding of each word.

Do yourself a favor and do not just give the shortest and simplest answer. Use the following example of anxiety: Instead of answering, "Anxiety is a mental state of being nervous," ask:

Is **anxiety** a medical condition? Who usually suffers from anxiety? Is anxiety related to other mental or medical conditions?

Who is at risk for developing **asthma**? How is it treated?

How is **gout** diagnosed? How is it medicated? Can it ever be medication induced?

How does **hypertension** affect other systems? What are the parameters for diagnosing it? How does it damage organs?

What are the causes of **hypothyroidism**? How does it affect medication administration?

What medications are used to treat **left heart failure (LHF)**? Which medications can contribute to the development of LHF?

Home Medications

☑ Self-Query: Possible Answers

Acetaminophen and hydrocodone (Anexsia) 7.5/650 orally 1–2 tabs every 4 hours as needed: this medication is a combination of acetaminophen (650 mg) and hydrocodone (7.5 mg). It is used for moderate to severe pain.

Albuterol (90 mcg) 2 puffs every 4 hours as needed: albuterol is a short-acting beta-2 adrenergic receptor agonist bronchodilator.

Allopurinol (Zyloprim) 300 mg orally daily: allopurinol decreases uric acid levels in the blood and urine by inhibiting the enzyme responsible for production of uric acid. It is used to treat gout.

Bumetanide (Bumex) 1 mg orally daily: bumetanide is a loop diuretic used to treat hypertension.

Buspirone 30 mg orally every 12 hours: buspirone, also known as BuSpar, is used as an antianxiety medicine. It affects chemicals in the brain that may become unbalanced and cause anxiety.

Digoxin 0.125 mg orally daily: digoxin is used to treat heart failure as well as atrial fibrillation. This individual suffers from both.

Levothyroxine 0.1 mg orally daily: Synthroid is a replacement for levothyroxine (T_4). Synthetic T_4 is identical to that produced in the thyroid gland.

Lisinopril 10 mg orally daily: lisinopril is an angiotensin-converting enzyme (ACE) inhibitor. It works in the kidneys and is prescribed for hypertension.

Mometasone 220 mcg daily inhalation: mometasone inhalation, also known as Nasonex nasal spray, is an anti-inflammatory corticosteroid used for seasonal allergic rhinitis.

Nebivolol 5 mg orally daily: nebivolol is a beta blocker. Beta blockers block beta-adrenergic receptors, which prevents adrenaline (epinephrine) from stimulating these receptors. Blocking the receptors slows the heart rate, reduces the force of contraction, and decreases blood pressure.

Omeprazole (Prilosec) 40 mg daily orally omeprazole decreases the amount of acid produced in the stomach. It is considered a proton pump inhibitor and is used to treat symptoms of gastroesophageal reflux disease (GERD) and other conditions caused by excess stomach acid.

Docusate/sennoside (Senokot-S) 2 pills daily as needed: docusate/sennoside is used to treat constipation and has a stool softener.

Warfarin 2 mg orally daily: warfarin, also known as Coumadin, is an anticoagulant and is used to prevent thrombosis and embolism.

Body Systems

☑ Self-Query: Possible Answers

Neurological

> Acetaminophen and hydrocodone 7.5/650 orally 2 tabs every 4 hours as needed
> Buspirone 30 mg orally every 12 hours

Cardiovascular

> Digoxin 0.125 mg orally daily
> Lisinopril 10 mg orally daily
> Bystolic 5 mg orally daily
> Warfarin 2 mg orally daily

Hematological

> Allopurinol 300 mg orally daily
> Warfarin 2 mg orally daily (In this case, it is used as a cardiac medication.)

Pulmonary

> Albuterol 90 mcg 2 puffs every 4 hours as needed
> May also alter heart rate

Gastrointestinal

> Omeprazole 40 mg daily orally
> Docusate/sennoside 2 pills daily as needed

Nutrition

> None specific

Genitourinary/renal

> Allopurinol 300 mg orally daily
> Bumetanide 1 mg orally daily
> Lisinopril 10 mg orally daily

Musculoskeletal

> Acetaminophen and hydrocodone 7.5/650 orally 1–2 tabs every 4 hours as needed

Endocrine

> Synthroid 0.1 mg orally daily

Integumentary

> None specific

Immune

> None specific; however, repeated inhalation of steroid may alter immunity.

Pain/comfort

> Acetaminophen and hydrocodone 7.5/650 orally 1–2 tabs every 4 hours as needed

38

Vocabulary

? Self-Query

Before attempting to work the case study, define each of the vocabulary words. Although the words may have several subheadings, it will give you a place to begin your inquiry.

Chemoreceptor trigger zone

_____

Chemotherapy

_____

Chemotherapy-induced nausea and vomiting (CINV)

_____

Decadron/Ativan/Benadryl (BAD) combination for nausea and vomiting

_____

Duodenal ulcer

_____

Palliative care

_____

Peptic ulcer

_____

You are the home health nurse making a visit to a 55-year-old female after a 5-day hospitalization for dehydration that followed her previous chemotherapy treatment for breast cancer.

Home Medications

Dexamethasone (Decadron) 1 mg every 12 hours

Docusate/sennoside (Senokot-S) 2 tabs every 6 hours until bowel movement for constipation not relieved by
magnesium

Dronabinol (Marinol) 5 mg orally every 2 hours as needed

Esomeprazole (Nexium) 20 mg orally daily

Magnesium 500 mg as needed for constipation

Morphine sulfate continuous release (MS Contin) 30 mg 3 tabs every 8 hours

Normal saline 1000 mL as needed for uncontrolled nausea and vomiting for 3 hours

Palonosetron (Aloxi) 0.25 mg IV (patient's daughter injects through PICC line)

⚕ Self-Query

Using a drug book or pharmacology text that contains the mechanism of action, unlabeled uses, and pharmacokinetics of medications, answer the following questions. Make answers specific to this scenario.

What do I know about these medications? Do I know the recommended dose of, the recommended route for, and the best time of day to give these medications? Do I know what lab results I need regarding each medication? Do I know the approved use of each medication? Do I know the most common diseases treated by the listed medications? Are any off-label uses approved for each drug?

Dexamethasone

_____

_____

Docusate/sennoside

_____

_____

Dronabinol

_____

_____

Esomeprazole

_____

_____

Magnesium

_____

_____

Morphine sulfate continuous release

_____

_____

Normal saline

_____

_____

Palonosetron

_____

_____

How do these medications interact with each other?

_____

_____

Why use docusate/sennoside and not plain sennoside?

_____

_____

What is the active ingredient in dronabinol?

_____

What other drugs are in the classification of palonosetron?

_____

_____

How long can a PICC line remain in place? How is it flushed?

_____

_____

Nursing Process

Self-Query

What nursing assessment should be done for each medication? What planning and implementation are needed in regard to each medication? How do I evaluate each medication's effectiveness?

Dexamethasone

_____

_____

Docusate/sennoside

_____

_____

Dronabinol

_____

_____

Esomeprazole

_____

_____

Magnesium

_____

_____

Morphine sulfate continuous release

_____

_____

Normal saline

_____

_____

Palonosetron

_____

_____

Develop two nursing diagnoses for this patient (NANDA).

_____

_____

Develop at least three patient outcomes (NOC).

_____

_____

_____

Develop at least three patient interventions (NIC).

_____

_____

_____

What nutritional issues need to be addressed?

_____

_____

Synopsis

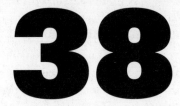

38

Because you can find answers to the self-queries in numerous texts, you will not find the answers to all of them here. However, you will find discussion of the individual case. The scenario relates to pain control during cancer treatment; therefore, purposefully look into the medication use and vocabulary as they relate to these factors.

Vocabulary

When reviewing the vocabulary words, you might want to ask several questions: who, what, where, when, why, and how. This should give you a much broader understanding of the word.

Do yourself a favor and do not just give the shortest and simplest answer. Use the following example of peptic ulcer: Instead of answering, "Peptic ulcers are ulcers located in the stomach," ask:

What medications can promote the development of a **peptic ulcer**? Who is at risk for peptic ulcers? Which medications are used to treat a peptic ulcer?

☑ Self-Query: Possible Answers

When defining the remainder of the vocabulary words, ask the following questions:

Where is the **chemoreceptor trigger zone**?

What medications are considered **chemotherapy**? Since all medications are chemicals and used for therapeutic reasons, in one sense all medications can be considered chemotherapy. However, when one thinks of chemotherapy, cancer is the first word that comes to the mind. Are all medications to be considered chemotherapy?

What causes **chemotherapy-induced nausea and vomiting (CINV)**? Which medications are most effective in this type of nausea? What is the treatment for CINV? Why is it important?

Break down the combination of **Decadron/Ativan/Benadryl (BAD)** used for nausea and vomiting and explain how it works. Keep in mind that this is a home health patient, and all this is prescribed for home administration.

What medications promote the development of a **duodenal ulcer**? Who is at risk for a duodenal ulcer? Which medications are used to treat a duodenal ulcer? How are duodenal and peptic ulcers different? What are the differences in the symptoms for each?

Who is eligible for **palliative care**? How is it different from hospice care?

Home Medications

☑ Self-Query: Possible Answers

Dexamethasone (Decadron) 1 mg every 12 hours: dexamethasone is a synthetic adrenocortical steroid prescribed to modify the body's immune responses. It decreases edema surrounding the tumor site. It is also used to decrease nausea.

Docusate/sennoside (Senokot-S) 2 tabs every 6 hours until bowel movement for constipation not relieved by magnesium: docusate/sennoside, from the senna plant, is used to treat constipation. Like nausea, constipation is commonly reported by cancer patients; one cause is pain medications. Always ask, "Have you had a bowel movement, and are you in pain?"

Dronabinol (Marinol) 5 mg orally every 2 hours as needed: dronabinol is a synthetic version of a naturally occurring compound known as THC, the active ingredient in marijuana. It is approved to treat nausea and vomiting associated with cancer chemotherapy. It is prescribed for individuals who have failed to respond to other conventional treatments. One positive side effect is increased appetite.

Esomeprazole (Nexium) 20 mg orally daily: esomeprazole is a proton pump inhibitor and blocks the production of H+ in the stomach. This in turn reduces gastric acid in the stomach.

Magnesium 500 mg as needed for constipation: magnesium, a gentle laxative, helps to prevent constipation by relaxing the colon. It is taken in the form of milk of magnesia.

Morphine sulfate continuous release (MS Contin) 30 mg (3 tabs) every 8 hours: morphine is an opioid used to treat moderate to severe pain.

Normal saline 1000 mL as needed for uncontrolled nausea and vomiting: this is infused in the home when the patient has uncontrolled nausea to prevent dehydration. If the nausea is not controlled by the administration of her numerous medications, she will be admitted to the hospital.

Palonosetron (Aloxi) 0.25 mg IV (patient's daughter injects through PICC line): palonosetron is an antiemetic. It alters the effect of serotonin receptors that play a part in CINV.

Case Study Inquiry

39

Vocabulary

☞ Self-Query

Before attempting to work the case study, define each of the vocabulary words. Although the words may have several subheadings, it will give you a place to begin your inquiry.

Bipolar disorder

_____

Dementia

_____

Hypothyroidism

_____

Major depression

_____

Neurotransmitters

_____

Obsessive-compulsive disorder (OCD)

_____

Omega-3 fatty acid

_____

You are caring for a 28-year-old female with a dual diagnosis of bipolar disorder and substance abuse. She has come to the office with her mother for a lithium level.

Home Medications

Cranberry capsules 2 daily
Docusate/sennoside (Senna-S) 2 tabs daily
Lithium 300 mg orally at bedtime (p.m.)
MVI 2 tabs daily
Pregabalin (Lyrica) 300 mg every 8 hours
Quetiapine (Seroquel) XR 300 mg at bedtime

☞ Self-Query

Using a drug book or pharmacology text that contains the mechanism of action, unlabeled uses, and pharmacokinetics of medications, answer the following questions. Make answers specific to this scenario.

What do I know about these medications? Do I know the recommended dose of, the recommended route for, and the best time of day to give these medications? Do I know what lab results I need regarding each medication? Do I know the approved use of each medication? Do I know the most common diseases treated by the listed medications? Are any off-label uses approved for each drug?

Cranberry capsules

_____

_____

Docusate/sennoside

_____

_____

Lithium

_____

_____

MVI

_____

_____

Pregabalin

_____

_____

Quetiapine

_____

_____

How do these medications interact with each other?

_____

_____

Why use docusate/sennoside and not plain sennoside?

_____

If the lithium was taken at 9 o'clock the previous night, when should the lithium level be drawn?

_____

Nursing Process

Self-Query

What nursing assessment should be done for each medication? What planning and implementation are needed in regard to each medication? How do I evaluate each medication's effectiveness?

Cranberry capsules

_____

_____

Docusate/sennoside

_____

_____

Lithium

_____

_____

MVI

_____

_____

Pregabalin

_____

_____

Quetiapine

_____

_____

Develop two nursing diagnoses for this patient (NANDA).

_____

_____

Develop at least three patient outcomes (NOC).

_____

_____

Develop at least three patient interventions (NIC).

_____

_____

What dietary issues need to be addressed?

_____

_____

Synopsis

39

Because you can find answers to the self-queries in numerous texts, you will not find the answers to all of them here. However, you will find discussion of the individual case. The scenario relates to medications used in mental illness and substance abuse. Therefore, purposefully look into the medication use and vocabulary as they relate to these factors.

Vocabulary

When reviewing the vocabulary words, you might want to ask several questions: who, what, where, when, why, and how. This should give you a much broader understanding of each word.

Do yourself a favor and do not just give the shortest and simplest answer. Use the following example of hypothyroidism: Instead of answering, "Bipolar disorder is a combination of high and low emotions," ask:

What is **bipolar disorder**? Who is at risk for bipolar disorder? How does it manifest itself? How is bipolar treated with medicines? How can anticonvulsant medications treat this disorder?

☑ Self-Query: Possible Answers

When defining the remainder of the vocabulary words, ask the following questions:

What is **dementia**? How it is medically treated? How is it different from depression and OCD?

What causes **hypothyroidism**? How is it treated? How does lithium alter the thyroid?

What is **major depression**? What are a few of the theorized causes? How is it treated medically?

What are **neurotransmitters**? What is their function?

What is **obsessive-compulsive disorder** (OCD)? What are its causes?

What does the "3" in **omega-3 fatty acid** refer to? How does it alter the clotting factors in the body? Can it be used as a mood stabilizer? How does it alter medication use in the liver?

Home Medications

☑ Self-Query: Possible Answers

Cranberry capsules 2 daily: cranberry capsules are used as a remedy for cystitis/UTI. Cranberries appear to make it difficult for bacteria to adhere to the bladder wall.

Docusate/sennoside (Senna-S) 2 tabs daily: docusate/sennoside is a combination of sennoside, a stimulant, and docusate, a stool softener. Stimulant laxatives, also known as contact laxatives, encourage bowel movements by causing muscle contractions of the intestinal wall. Stool softeners encourage bowel movements by drawing liquids into the stool and preventing dry, hard stool masses. Stool softeners allow a soft movement without straining. Adding a softener assists in decreasing regularly hard stools.

Lithium 300 mg orally at bedtime (p.m.): lithium is also known as Eskalith. People may develop lithium toxicity because the effective dose is close to the toxic dose. It is mandatory that healthcare providers obtain blood tests to measure the lithium blood levels. Dosage is based on levels. The blood test for lithium levels is taken at a specific time, usually 8–12 hours after the last dose. This patient's nightly dose is taken at 9:00 p.m. Blood level was drawn at 9 a.m. and was 0.8, which is therapeutic for her. This is a case of the dosage being individualized. The patient began with 300 mg twice a day; however, she developed lithium toxicity and was moved to 300 mg at night only.

MVI 2 tabs daily: prevention of nutritional deficiencies with vitamins, herbs, and supplements is a popular approach to maintaining good health. This individual's mother wants her to take to supplements because she thinks they help stabilize her daughter's mood and prevent mood swings. In addition, her daughter does not have a proper intake of nutrients.

Pregabalin (Lyrica) 300 mg every 8 hours: pregabalin is considered an anticonvulsant. It is approved to treat diabetic neuropathy and postherpetic nerve pain following shingles, and fibromyalgia. It works by slowing down impulses in the brain. It is also being used in patients with bipolar disorder, with some success.

Quetiapine (Seroquel) XR 300 mg at bedtime: quetiapine is an antipsychotic medication used to control the manic episodes in bipolar disorder and to assist in stabilizing moods. It alters dopamine, serotonin, and histamine-1 receptors.

Nursing Process

☑ Self-Query: Possible Answers

Lithium and drug issues: Nonsteroidal anti-inflammatory drugs (NSAIDs) reduce the kidneys' ability to eliminate lithium and lead to elevated levels of lithium. Aspirin does not appear to affect lithium concentrations in the blood. Diuretics that act at the distal renal tubule can increase blood concentrations of lithium. Diuretics that act at the proximal tubule are more likely to reduce blood concentrations of lithium. Diuretics such as furosemide seem to have no effect on lithium concentrations in blood. ACE inhibitors seem to increase the risk of developing lithium toxicity because they increase lithium reabsorb ion and reduce the excretion.

Lithium and diet issues: Individuals with mania are often treated with lithium. Sodium and caffeine intake can affect lithium levels in the blood, and intake of these should not suddenly be increased or decreased. Weight gain can occur in response to some antidepressant medications and lithium. If the preceding medications are needed, the process of individualizing the dose will have to be adjusted.

Regarding diet education, individuals taking lithium should maintain a consistent intake of sodium (found in table salt and other food additives) and caffeine in the diet. Restricting sodium for any reason causes less lithium to be excreted in the urine, and blood lithium levels rise. If an individual increases caffeine intake, more lithium is excreted in the urine, and blood levels of lithium fall.

Case Study Inquiry

40

Your instructor wants you to have an educated idea of what the medical diagnosis for a patient might be after reviewing a medication list. Your instructor only allows you to review the medications of three patients you will care for with a preceptor the next day, and not the charts, to find the diagnosis. You will be given the medical diagnosis on the day you care for the patient.

Patient #1

Patient #1 is an admission with the following medications:

Aspirin (Ecotrin) 325 mg orally daily

Cefpodoxime (Vantin) 200 mg twice a day orally

Chlordiazepoxide hydrochloride (Librium) 25 mg 3 times a day orally

Furosemide (Lasix) 40 mg every day orally

Lorazepam (Ativan) 1 mg orally: 1–2 every 2–4 hours orally as needed

Nitro paste 1 inch every 6 hours topically

Oxazepam (Serax) 15 mg orally every 12 hours

Potassium chloride 20 mEq every day orally

Thiamine hydrochloride (B1) 100-mg tab daily

Self-Query

Use a pharmacology, pathophysiology, and assessment text to develop a plan of care. Use NANDA/ NOC/NIC.

What lab results will you review?

_____

_____

What diagnostic exams will be needed?

_____

_____

Patient #2

Patient #2 is a new admit with the following medication orders:

Albuterol and ipratropium (Combivent) inhaled 18 mcg 2–3 puffs daily

Aspirin (ASA) 81 mg orally with lunch

Atorvastatin (Lipitor) 20 mg orally daily

Celecoxib (Celebrex) 200 mg orally daily

Clopidogrel (Plavix) 75 mg orally daily

Fluticasone and salmeterol (Advair) 250/50 (patient has the prescription but never filled it)

Glipizide 10 mg orally daily

Guaifenesin 200 mg every 12 hours

Iron 27 mg orally daily

Metformin 500 mg orally twice daily

Pantoprazole 40 mg orally daily

Vancomycin 1 g every 24 hours

Self-Query

Use a pharmacology, pathophysiology, and assessment text to develop a plan of care. Use NANDA/ NOC/NIC.

What lab results will you review?

_____

_____

What diagnostic exams will be needed?

_____

_____

Patient #3

Patient #3 is a new admit with the following orders:

Albuterol (Proventil) 2.5 mg/3 mL every 4–6 hours

Ceftriaxone (Rocephin) 1 g every 12 hours

Esomeprazole (Nexium) 40 mg orally before lunch

Furosemide (Lasix) 40 mg orally before breakfast

Insulin glargine (Lantus) 40 units subcutaneously at bedtime

Nebivolol (Bystolic) 5 mg orally daily

Potassium chloride (K-Dur) 20 mEq taken with furosemide

Prednisone 5 mg orally daily

Theophylline (Slo-Bid) 200 mg orally twice a day every 12 hours

Tramadol (Ultram) 100 mg extended release daily

Allergies

Ceftazidime (Fortaz)

Self-Query

Use a pharmacology, pathophysiology, and assessment text to develop a plan of care. Use NANDA/ NOC/NIC.

What lab results will you review?

_____

_____

What diagnostic exams will be needed?

_____

_____

Find the classifications of these medications and decide if any are duplicates, and why?

_____

_____

Synopsis

40

Many students say, "Why do I need to know medications? I can look them up on the unit before I give them if I am not sure." The answer to that is obvious to most of us who have been given five or six patients at one time—patients who, unfortunately, may have more than 10 medications due at once. It is not possible to look up that many medications on that many patients and have the medications given on time, not to mention that numerous other issues are usually playing out at the same time (phone calls, patient and family requests, healthcare providers asking questions, and assisting other nurses). Throw an occasional new admission or code situation into the mix, and you now have the picture. Also remember that most people do not have just one issue; a patient may be admitted for one problem and have numerous other issues.

Example: An 87-year-old individual who has a pacemaker malfunction (cardiac), develops vertigo and syncope (neurological), and falls and fractures her shoulder (orthopedic) can be a challenge because she will be on several different medications and seen by numerous healthcare providers. She also has special geriatric considerations.

The scenario relates to team leading for three patients and their medications. You are the oncoming nurse for the 7 a.m. to 7 p.m. rotation.

Patient #1

☑ Self-Query: Possible Answers

Patient #1 was admitted around 4 a.m. You rule out a hip fracture from a fall.

Cefpodoxime (Vantin) 200 mg twice a day orally

You need to know:

> What is the patient's white blood cell count and what were the results of any cultures that have been collected? Why was it prescribed?
> Is it still needed?
> Are cefpodoxime and cefazolin (Ancef) in the same family of drugs?

Furosemide (Lasix) 40 mg every day orally

You need to know:

> Potassium level
> Blood pressure

Nitro paste 1 inch every 6 hours topically

You need to know:

> Blood pressure

Potassium chloride 20 mEq every day orally

You need to know:

> Potassium level
> Blood pressure

Thiamine

You need to know:

Thiamine levels
Assess for anemia

The patient is requesting pain medications, and her family is upset. They believe that she is not being cared for because she has a history of alcohol abuse. Make sure you are aware of the reasons that all the medications are given. Discuss with your group how additional addictive substances (PCA pump of morphine and acetaminophen/oxycodone [Percocet]) may play out in this individual's care.

Patient #2

☑ Self-Query: Possible Answers

Postoperative day 1 for revision of right knee surgery infection.

Albuterol and ipratropium (Combivent) inhaled 18 mcg 2–3 puffs daily

Respiratory therapy has to be notified for breathing treatment.

Aspirin (ASA) 81 mg orally with lunch

You need to know if the individual stopped the drug 5 days before surgery. If so, when does the healthcare provider want it resumed?

Atorvastatin (Lipitor) 20 mg orally daily

Liver panel profile results are needed. When was the individual's most recent cholesterol level taken?

Clopidogrel (Plavix) 75 mg orally daily

You need to assess for bleeding because this medication was not stopped before surgery.

Glipizide 10 mg orally daily

Before meals and at bedtime glucose monitoring need to be scheduled. Is a sliding scale needed while the individual is in the hospital?

Iron 27 mg orally daily

Because of past iron deficiency, the patient will have Hct/Hgb/ PT/INR daily until discharge.

Metformin 500 mg orally twice daily

Before meals and at bedtime glucose monitoring need to be scheduled. Is a sliding scale needed while the individual is in the hospital?

Vancomycin 1 gram every 24 hours

Does this need to be continued after knee surgery?
The patient has been on vancomycin for 2 weeks. Does a peak and trough need to be drawn for the vancomycin?
Can vancomycin be easily interchanged between oral and IV administration? Explain the answer you give.

Postop day 1 reveals a Hgb of 8.2 (you know that this as the iron-containing protein that bonds with oxygen, allowing the red blood cells to transport oxygen throughout the body). Postop day 1 also reveals a Hct of 29.8 (you know this as the portion of blood consisting of red blood cells). The physician tells you to give 2 units of packed red blood cells. The individual has auto blood (the donation of one's own blood products before surgery and reinfused after surgery as needed). You now have the task of blood infusion, in addition to other duties (it is only 8:30 a.m.).

Reassess for bleeding because anticoagulants were not stopped prior to surgery. The patient requests pain medication (2 tabs acetaminophen/oxycodone) before attending joint class. You know that this needs to be given now to be in effect for the class in 1 hour.

The following medications are ordered after surgery:

Carisoprodol (Soma) every 6 hours orally for muscle spasms
Ketorolac (Toradol) 10 mg every 6 hours IV
Morphine 2–4 mg every 3 hours as needed for pain
Ondansetron (Zofran) 2 mg IV every 4 hours as needed for nausea

Discuss why these medications were ordered and the nursing interventions for them.

Patient #3

☑ Self-Query: Possible Answers

Patient #3 is postoperative from back surgery and will be on the unit in 1 hour.

Pharmacy calls asking for confirmation on allergy because ceftazidime (Fortaz) and ceftriaxone (Rocephin) are in the same family. The patient's family is asking about routine medications. Because the patient did not have a.m. meds, they want the blood sugar and blood pressure checked now. Because of the diabetes history, you will be placing the individual on insulin while in the hospital. You will need the morning glucose value to see if any coverage is needed. Respiratory therapy needs consult. Tramadol (Ultram) is stopped until discharge. The following medications are ordered after surgery:

Carisoprodol (Soma) every 6 hours orally for muscle spasms
Ketorolac (Toradol) 10 mg every 6 hours IV
Morphine 2–4 mg every 3 hours as needed for pain
Ondansetron (Zofran) 2 mg IV every 4 hours as needed for nausea
Vancomycin 1 g first dose (then have pharmacy dose)

Are the IV medications compatible?

41

Vocabulary

Self-Query

Before attempting to work the case study, define each of the vocabulary words. Although the words may have several subheadings, it will give you a place to begin your inquiry.

Acute renal failure
_____

Angiotensin-converting enzyme
_____

Bisphosphonate
_____

Chronic renal failure
_____

End-stage renal failure
_____

High-ceiling (loop) diuretics
_____

Osteoarthritis (OA)
_____

Osteoporosis
_____

Type I diabetes
_____

Type II diabetes
_____

Your new patient is a 70-year-old African American female discharged 8 weeks ago from your unit after recovering from left-sided congestive heart failure. She is slightly dyspneic and has 2+ edema in her lower extremities. She also reveals an S_3 heart sound. Her blood pressure is 140/90 and heart rate is 90 with irregular pulse.

Home Medications

Aspirin (ASA) 81 mg orally daily

Bumetanide (Bumex) 1 mg orally daily

Calcium carbonate (Tums) 2 chewable tabs orally daily (began after last admission)

Digoxin 0.125 mg orally daily

Ibandronate (Boniva) 3 mg IV every 3 months (first dose 2½ months ago)

Pioglitazone (Actos) 15 mg orally daily (added in last 4 weeks)

Potassium chloride (K-Dur) 40 mEq orally day

Ramipril (Altace) 5 mg orally daily

Zaleplon (Sonata) 5 mg orally at bedtime

Self-Query

Give the classification of each medication below and explain how its effectiveness is measured. Be sure to also answer any additional questions for each medication.

Aspirin: How do we want it to affect this patient?

_____

_____

Bumetanide: What is the mechanism of action in this medication?

_____

_____

Calcium carbonate

_____

_____

Digoxin: How does it work?

_____

_____

Ibandronate

_____

_____

Pioglitazone: What is an adverse side effect of this medication, other than hypoglycemia?

_____

_____

Potassium chloride

_____

_____

Ramipril: What happens when this medication classification elevates bradykinin? What happens when this classification reduces angiotensin II? What are two examples of these adverse effects?

_____

_____

Zaleplon: Why is it used in this patient? Is this a drug that can be given after midnight? (Explain your answer.)

_____

_____

Body Systems

Self-Query

Be prepared to defend your answers.

Can I place each medication under the body system that it commonly affects?

Neurological
_____

Cardiovascular
_____

Hematological
_____

Pulmonary
_____

Gastrointestinal
_____

Nutrition
_____

Genitourinary/renal
_____

Musculoskeletal
_____

Endocrine
_____

Integumentary
_____

Immune
_____

Pain/comfort
_____

Nursing Process

Self-Query

Using a drug book or pharmacology text that contains the mechanism of action, unlabeled uses, and pharmacokinetics for medications, answer the following questions. Make answers specific to this scenario.

Create a possible medical history and then match the present medications to the appropriate medical history.

_____

_____

_____

Reviewing the patient's history, you see that she was changed from chlorothiazide 25-mg tabs to bumetanide 1 mg. How are these medications similar? How are these medications different? What does the use of these medications tell us about the function of the kidneys?

_____

_____

The patient states that she has followed her diet and fluid restrictions religiously but continues to retain fluid. Which of her medications is possibly causing the fluid retention?

_____

Does it matter when she takes the medications in regard to each other? Which medication needs to be taken as far as possible from the other medications?

_____

Physician Orders

The physician orders the following lab work; some of the results are available.

Creatinine clearance (When should these results be ready? How is this test collected?)

BUN 30

Creatinine 1.2

Blood glucose 280

Hemoglobin 9.2

Hematocrit 30.8

Potassium 5.0

Liver function test

Digoxin level 0.1

Serum albumin 2.1

You call the admitting physician with the list of medications and lab values, and after reading off the list, you receive the following orders. Be able to discuss why the orders were given.

Stop ramipril 5 mg orally daily (Don't we need this for the blood pressure?)

Digoxin level returns and is 0.1 (Is this therapeutic?)

Stop digoxin 0.125 mg orally daily (Don't we need this for the dysrhythmia?)

Begin verapamil 80 mg orally every 8 hours

Stop pioglitazone 15 mg orally daily, monitor blood sugar every a.m. (Don't we need this for the type II DM?)

Stop bumetanide 1 mg orally daily, change to furosemide (Lasix) 40 mg IV now and daily

Aspirin 81 mg orally daily

See when ibandronate is due and give if needed; ibandronate 3 mg IV every 3 months

Calcium carbonate 2 chewable tabs orally daily

IV normal saline at 50 mL/hr, strict intake and output

❓ Self-Query

Match the lab work above to the patient's original medications and be able to discuss your choices.

_____

_____

_____

What classification is verapamil? What is the mechanism of action in this medication? How do we measure effectiveness?

_____

_____

What classification is furosemide? What is the mechanism of action in this medication? How do we measure effectiveness?

_____

_____

Which medications, past and present, are affected by the potassium level?

_____

Which medications are affected by low albumin levels? How does a low albumin level interfere with medications being used in the body?

_____

Are ibandronate and furosemide compatible, and can they be infused in the same IV line? What is the advantage of infusing the two medications in relation to oral administration? What are the infusion guidelines for the two medications? Explain your answers to these three questions.

_____

_____

Nursing Process

Self-Query

What nursing assessment should be done for each medication? What planning and implementation do I need to do in regard to each medication? How do I evaluate each medication's effectiveness? How do these prescribed medications work?

Aspirin

_____

_____

Calcium carbonate

_____

_____

Furosemide

_____

_____

Ibandronate

_____

_____

Normal saline

_____

Verapamil

_____

_____

Develop two nursing diagnoses for this patient (NANDA) in regard to the medications.

_____

_____

Develop at least three patient outcomes (NOC) in regard to the medications.

_____

_____

_____

Develop at least three patient interventions (NIC) in regard to the medications.

_____

_____

_____

What dietary issues need to be addressed?

_____

_____

Medical History

Left-sided heart failure
Type II diabetes
Hypertension
Atrial fibrillation
Renal insufficiency
Osteoporosis

Synopsis

41

Because you can find answers to the self-queries in numerous texts, you will not find the answers to all of them here. However, you will find discussion of the individual case. Therefore, purposefully look into the medication use and vocabulary as they relate to these factors.

Vocabulary

When reviewing the vocabulary words, you might want to ask several questions: who, what, where, when, why, and how. This should give you a much broader understanding of each word.

Do yourself a favor and do not just give the shortest and simplest answer. The following questions are to be used as a guide. Apply the following example, bisphosphonate, to all the vocabulary words. Instead of answering, "Bisphosphonates are drugs that prevent bone loss," ask:

What is a **bisphosphonate**? Who uses bisphosphonate? How are bisphosphonates connected to osteonecrosis of the jaw?

☑ Self-Query: Possible Answers

When defining the remainder of the vocabulary words, ask the following questions:

Why conduct an assessment for **acute renal failure** in a patient with bone disease?

What is the **angiotensin-converting enzyme (ACE)**? Where does it work?

Who is at risk for **chronic renal failure**? How is it treated?

How is **end-stage renal failure** treated?

Which diuretics are considered **high-ceiling (loop) diuretics**? Why do they continue to work even in renal insufficiency?

What is **osteoarthritis (OA)**? Who is at risk for OA? How does a bisphosphonate treat OA?

Who is at risk for **osteoporosis**? How is it treated?

What is the difference between **type I diabetes** and **type II diabetes**?

Home Medications

☑ Self-Query: Possible Answers

Aspirin (ASA) 81 mg orally daily (for antiplatelet possible history of MI/CVA/TIA): acetylsalicylic acid can be used as an analgesic, antipyretic, and anti-inflammatory. It is considered an NSAID. In this case, it is used as an antiplatelet medication; antiplatelet agents block the formation of blood clots (thrombus formation) by preventing the clumping of platelets (aggregation).

Bumetanide (Bumex) 1 mg orally daily: bumetanide is a high-ceiling (loop) diuretic. It is used for hypertension/renal disease/edema. 1 mg of bumetanide has shown the same potency as approximately 40 mg furosemide. It is used to manage edema in heart failure; it may be used with an antihypertensive in the treatment of hypertension.

Calcium carbonate (Tums) 2 chewable tabs orally daily: patient began using after last admission for calcium replacement/indigestion. Calcium carbonate is chalk. Because of the age of the individual, this may not be absorbed by her body. Her calcium level was not low, so she opted for the less expensive route as a supplement.

Digoxin 0.125 mg orally daily: cardiac glycosides. Digoxin slows the heart rate and increases contractions and is used mostly for atrial fibrillation and flutter; it also may be used in patients with heart failure.

Ibandronate (Boniva) 3 mg IV every 3 months (first dose 2½ months ago for osteoporosis): bisphosphonates slow or stop the natural process that dissolves bone tissue, resulting in maintained or increased bone density and strength. This may prevent the development of osteoporosis. If osteoporosis has already developed, slowing the rate of bone thinning reduces the risk of broken bones. Bisphosphonates may be taken by men or women and are commonly used for the prevention and treatment of osteoporosis. If bisphosphonates are prescribed, calcium and vitamin D supplements should be prescribed as well, and the patient should undergo a kidney assessment.

Pioglitazone (Actos) 15 mg orally daily (added in last 4 weeks for type II diabetes): pioglitazone is used to treat type II diabetes; it alters the body's cells to use glucose more effectively. Side effects include feeling short of breath with mild exertion, edema or swelling, and rapid weight gain.

Potassium chloride (K-Dur) 40 mEq orally day: potassium chloride is a potassium supplement.

Ramipril (Altace) 5 mg orally daily (for hypertension): ramipril is an ACE inhibitor used as an anti-hypertension medication. ACE is responsible for producing the chemical angiotensin II. Angiotensin II causes arteries, including the arteries of the heart, to contract, thereby narrowing the arteries and elevating blood pressure. ACE inhibitors reduce the production of angiotensin II, thereby relaxing and dilating arteries. Blood pressure is decreased, and kidney function may be improved. Two common side effects of ramipril are cough and angioedema.

Zapelon (Sonata) 5 mg orally at bedtime (for insomnia): zaleplon is a sedative used to treat insomnia. This medication causes relaxation to help patients fall asleep and stay asleep. Zaleplon possesses anticonvulsant, anxiolytic, and hypnotic properties. It assists this patient in falling asleep, and if she doesn't use it, she wakes up several times during the night.

Body Systems

☑ Self-Query: Possible Answers

Neurological

> Zaleplon

Cardiovascular

> Potassium chloride
> Aspirin
> Bumetanide
> Digoxin

Hematological

> Calcium carbonate
> Aspirin
> Ibandronate

Pulmonary

> None specific

Gastrointestinal

Some will place calcium carbonate here. This is a situation in which it alters gastrointestinal lining but is actually used for its calcium content. This is a case of drugs not being selective.

Nutrition

Pioglitazone
Review the mechanism of action and note that it actually could be placed under any of the headings.

Genitourinary/renal

Bumetanide

Musculoskeletal

Ibandronate
Calcium carbonate

Endocrine

Some may place pioglitazone here; however, examine its mechanism of action.

Integumentary

None specific

Immune

None specific

Pain/comfort

The patient did not report using any drugs for pain and comfort. However, she should be asked about use of over-the-counter medications such as Tylenol.

Nursing Process

☑ Self-Query: Possible Answers

Chlorothiazide changed to bumetanide: chlorothiazide is a thiazide diuretic. The woman had been taking this medication for many years before it was stopped. The provider who prescribed this medication used chlorothiazide for two purposes at first: (1) The patient had developed hypertension and needed a diuretic, and (2) the provider at that time also thought that it would promote calcium retention and slow the patient's development of osteoporosis.

When she developed renal insufficiency, the thiazide no longer worked.

Bumetanide is a high-ceiling (loop) diuretic. The healthcare provider stopped the chlorothiazide several years ago and prescribed the bumetanide for the following reasons: (1) The patient's hypertension was not controlled by the thiazide diuretic; (2) her cardiac status deteriorated because of her hypertension-causing left ventricular failure; and (3) her creatinine and BUN revealed renal insufficiency, and only the loop diuretics are effective in this case. Both medications can cause potassium loss.

Pioglitazone has been shown to cause edema in individuals with mild heart disease or any problems with their kidneys. Calcium carbonate used as a calcium replacement is also given for gastric hyperacidity; it should not be taken within 2 hours of any other medications. Calcium carbonate can cause digoxin toxicity.

The creatinine clearance compares creatinine levels in the urine with the creatinine level in the blood. Urine is collected for 24 hours in a special container, and blood is drawn at the end of the 24-hour period.

BUN 30—renal (bumetanide)

Creatinine 1.2—renal (bumetanide)

Remember the pharmacokinetics of each medication (absorption/distribution/metabolism/excretion)

Blood glucose 280 metabolic—pioglitazone

Hemoglobin 9.2—actually, this level is surprising because the patient has renal insufficiency and edema.

Hematocrit 30.8 (see hemoglobin)

Potassium 5.0—renal (bumetanide)

Electrolyte (potassium chloride)

Liver function test—this will give us an idea of how well she is metabolizing the medications. Remember the pharmacokinetics of each medication (absorption/distribution/metabolism/excretion).

Digoxin level 0.1—cardiac (Digoxin). This medication is highly altered by hyper/hypokalemia.

Serum albumin 2.1—this gives us an idea of how well all the medications are being distributed. Remember the pharmacokinetics of each medication (absorption/distribution/metabolism/excretion).

Ramipril was stopped because of the patient's hyperkalemia (ACE inhibitors have this side effect in renal insufficiency).

Digoxin, although an adequate medication, has been replaced with more effective and less troublesome medications. Her level was not therapeutic.

Pioglitazone was stopped because of its connection to her edema.

Begin verapamil 80 mg orally every 8 hours. Verapamil is classified as a calcium channel blocker. It relaxes the muscles of the heart and blood vessels. Verapamil was prescribed to treat her hypertension and atrial fibrillation.

See bumetanide for the classification and mechanism of action. However, the furosemide IV is in the hospital formulary and is given to the patient. The IV route is much quicker; it works in 5 minutes and lasts around 2 hours.

Aspirin 81 mg orally daily—this was continued.

Ibandronate 3 mg IV every 3 months—this was not due.

Calcium carbonate 2 chewable tabs orally daily—this was continued.

IV normal saline at 50 mL/hr strict intake and output.

IV administration bypasses barriers to absorption—directly into circulation. Ibandronate is administered intravenously over 15–30 seconds. Furosemide should be infused no more than 4 mg/mL.

Dietary: Sodium restrictions and diabetic considerations.

Case Study Inquiry

42

Vocabulary

? Self-Query

Before attempting to work the case study, define the vocabulary words. Although the words may have several subheadings, it will give you a place to begin your inquiry.

Glucagon
_____

Glycemic index
_____

Hypoglycemia
_____

Insulin resistance
_____

Lactic acidosis
_____

Lipodystrophies
_____

Type I diabetes mellitus
_____

Type II diabetes mellitus
_____

Recent History

Your have been Mr. Tripp's home health nurse for 3 months, caring for a wound infection related to a hip replacement. He has received his last dose of daptomycin (Cubicin) IV through his PICC line and now begins his oral prescription for the same medication. He was to be discharged from home health services today; however, when you arrive at the house, his wife states that he has been acting "different."

? Self-Query

What classification is Cubicin? What is the mechanism of action in this medication? How do we measure effectiveness? Does this medication require a trough? Does this medication require a peak?
_____
_____

What are the differences between Cubicin and vancomycin? (Discuss two.)
_____
_____

Physical Assessment Findings

You assess Mr. Tripp and find the following:

Neurological Assessment

Drowsy; pupils equal, round and reactive to light

Slight jerking of his extremities noted

Cardiovascular and Hematological Assessment

S_1S_2 apical pulse 120

Blood pressure 90/50, capillary refill at 3 seconds

Pulmonary Assessment

Lungs clear

Gastrointestinal Assessment

His wife states that he has been "sick at his stomach but did not vomit."

No history of diabetes, 250 pounds, 5'10" tall

Genitourinary Assessment

Bedside urinal full of light-colored urine

Musculoskeletal Assessment

Minimal movement

Endocrine Assessment

No history of DM

No chemstrips or glucometer in the home

Integumentary Assessment

Present PICC line without problems

Skin warm, face is flushed

Immune Assessment

No palpable lymph nodes

No inflammation noted in joints

Pain/Comfort Assessment

Speech slow, denies pain

States that he is just a little tired and wants to rest

Home Medications

Review the patient's home medications and attempt to determine his past medical history.

Aspirin (ASA) 81 mg orally daily

Calcium carbonate (Os-Cal) with vitamin D 2 tabs orally daily

Cyclobenzaprine (Flexeril) 10 mg orally 3 times a day

Magnesium hydroxide (Milk of Magnesia) 30 mL every morning

Potassium chloride (K-Dur) 40 mEq orally daily

Saw palmetto 1 dose every morning

Torsemide (Demadex) 10 mg orally daily

Verapamil 240 mg orally daily

Vitamin C 1 g orally daily

Self-Query

Using a drug book or pharmacology text that contains the mechanism of action, unlabeled uses, and pharmacokinetics of medications, answer the following questions. Make answers specific to this scenario.

Using the list you created of the patient's possible past medical history, match the medications to the appropriate medical diagnosis history.

_____

_____

_____

Allergies

None

Body Systems

Self-Query

Be prepared to defend your answers.

Can I place each medication under the body system that it commonly affects?

Neurological

_____

Cardiovascular

_____

Hematological

_____

Pulmonary

_____

Gastrointestinal

_____

Nutrition

_____

Genitourinary/renal

_____

Musculoskeletal

_____

Endocrine

_____

Integumentary

_____

Immune

_____

Pain/comfort

_____

After your assessment, you call the primary care provider and discuss your findings. She requests that you send the patient to the emergency department.

Emergency Department Lab and Assessment Findings
Neurological Assessment

Drowsy; pupils bilaterally equal, round, and reactive to light

Slight jerking of his extremities noted

Cardiovascular and Hematological Assessment

S_1S_2, sinus tachycardia 120 per monitor

Blood pressure 90/50, capillary refill at 3 seconds

ECG reveals peaked T waves

Pulmonary Assessment

Lungs clear

Gastrointestinal Assessment

Nauseated

No history of diabetes

Weight 250 pounds

Height 5'10"

Glucose monitor reads HHH

Serum glucose 950

Potassium 2.9

Sodium 130

Genitourinary Assessment

Physician requests indwelling catheter

In 1 hour, 500 mL light-colored urine returned

No ketones noted in urine

Musculoskeletal Assessment

Minimal movement

Endocrine Assessment

No history of DM

Integumentary Assessment

Present PICC line without problems

Skin warm, face is flushed

Immune Assessment

No palpable lymph nodes

No inflammation noted in joints

Pain/Comfort Assessment

Speech slow, denies pain

States that he is just a little tired and wants to rest

Physician Orders

The patient is admitted to ICU with following orders:

Pulmonary artery catheter is inserted.

  Vital signs, neurological assessment, and wedge reading every 15 minutes $\times$ 4
  Vital signs, neurological assessment, and wedge reading every 30 minutes $\times$ 4
  Vital signs, neurological assessment, and wedge reading every hour $\times$ 4
  Then, assessment every 4 hours

Begin hourly serum values of potassium, magnesium, and glucose

IV 0.45% saline 2 liters over 2 hours in PICC line

  Then infuse 0.45% saline @ 150 mL/hr
  IV regular insulin 0.15/kg now
  IV insulin 0.1 unit/kg/hr continuous infusion
  Decrease insulin drip to 0.05 unit/kg/hr when blood glucose is 300
  When serum glucose is 300, convert 0.45% saline to $D_5$1/2 saline
  When serum glucose is 200, stop IV insulin; use subcutaneous insulin per protocol

☀ Self-Query

What nursing assessment should be done regarding the infusion order?

_____

_____

How will rehydration affect the neurological status of this person?

_____

_____

Why the use of 0.45% saline?

_____

What planning and implementation do I need to do in regard to each medication?

_____

_____

How do I evaluate the effectiveness of the fluid and insulin?

_____

_____

How do these prescribed therapies work?

_____

_____

Why are the potassium and magnesium given along with the glucose?

_____

Develop two nursing diagnoses for this patient (NANDA) in regard to the medications.

_____

_____

Develop at least three patient outcomes (NOC) in regard to the medications.

_____

_____

_____

Develop at least three patient interventions (NIC) in regard to the medications.

_____

_____

_____

What dietary issues need to be addressed?

_____

_____

Follow-up

The patient recovers and is sent home with the following medications:

Aspirin (ASA) 81 mg orally daily

Calcium (Os-Cal) with vitamin D 2 tabs orally daily

Cyclobenzaprine (Flexeril) 10 mg orally 3 times a day

Magnesium hydroxide (Milk of Magnesia) 30 mL as needed

Metformin 500 mg orally twice daily

Potassium chloride (K-Dur) 40 mEq orally daily

Rosiglitazone (Avandia) 4 mg orally daily

Torsemide (Demadex) 10 mg orally daily

Verapamil 240 mg orally daily

Self-Query

What planning and implementation do I need to do in regard to rosiglitazone?

_____

_____

What planning and implementation do I need to do in regard to metformin?

_____

_____

How do I evaluate their effectiveness?

_____

_____

How do these prescribed therapies work?

_____

_____

What do these two new medications reveal about what happened to the patient?

_____

_____

Develop two nursing diagnoses for this patient (NANDA) in regard to the new medications.

_____

_____

Develop at least three patient outcomes (NOC) in regard to the new medications.

_____

_____

Develop at least three patient interventions (NIC) in regard to the new medications.

_____

_____

What dietary/life skills need to be addressed?

_____

_____

Synopsis

42

Because you can find answers to the self-queries in numerous texts, you will not find the answers to all of them here. However, you will find discussion of the individual case. The scenario relates to medications used in hyperglycemic hyperosmolar nonketotic syndrome (HHNS); therefore, purposefully look into the medication use and vocabulary as they relate to these factors.

Vocabulary

When reviewing the vocabulary words, you might want to ask several questions: who, what, where, when, why, and how. This should give you a much broader understanding of each word.

Do yourself a favor and do not just give the shortest and simplest answer. The following questions are to be used as a guide. Apply the following example, glycemic index, to all the vocabulary words. Instead of answering, "Glycemic index measures the effect of carbohydrates on blood sugar levels," ask:

What is an individual's **glycemic index**? Why is it measured?

☑ Self-Query: Possible Answers

When defining the remainder of the vocabulary words, ask the following questions:

Where is **glucagon** stored? What does it do?

What are symptoms of **hypoglycemia**? How is it treated?

What is **insulin resistance**? What causes it?

What causes **lactic acidosis**? Why are diabetics at risk?

What causes **lipodystrophies**? Who is at risk for developing lipodystrophies?

What is the physical appearance of an individual with **type I diabetes mellitus**? How is this disease medicated?

What is the physical appearance of an individual with **type II diabetes mellitus**? How is this disease medicated?

Recent History

☑ Self-Query: Possible Answers

Daptomycin (Cubicin) is a relatively new antibiotic classification. It was prescribed for this individual for a wound infection related to his hip replacement. Daptomycin binds to bacterial membranes and causes membrane death. Doses are calculated and range from 4 to 12 mg/kg in once-a-day dosing. His dose was 4 mg/kg over 30 minutes every 24 hours. This medication is compatible with 0.9% sodium chloride or lactated Ringer's injection. It is not compatible with dextrose solutions. It appears to be effective against most bacterial infections. It is different from vancomycin in that it does not require a peak or trough.

Home Medications

☑ **Self-Query: Possible Answers**

Aspirin (ASA) 81 mg orally daily: myocardial infarction, brain infarction, transient ischemic attack (TIA)

Verapamil 240 mg orally daily: hypertension, irregular rhythm

Calcium carbonate (Os-Cal) with vitamin D 2 tabs orally daily: osteoarthritis

Cyclobenzaprine (Flexeril) 10 mg orally three times a day: musculoskeletal

Magnesium hydroxide (Milk of Magnesia) 30 mL every morning: over-the-counter self-medication for constipation

Potassium chloride (K-Dur) 40 mEq orally daily: potassium replacement (on diuretic)

Saw palmetto one dose every morning: herbal/alternative over-the-counter for prostate health

Torsemide (Demadex) 10 mg orally daily; hypertension, heart failure

Vitamin C 1 gram orally daily: vitamin

Body Systems

☑ **Self-Query: Possible Answers**

Neurological

   Cyclobenzaprine

Cardiovascular

   Verapamil
   Aspirin
   Potassium chloride
   Torsemide

Hematological

   Aspirin
   Potassium chloride
   Calcium with vitamin D

Pulmonary

   None specific

Gastrointestinal

   Magnesium hydroxide
   Be aware of aspirin's alterations to this system. Also be aware of the interaction of this system with calcium with vitamin D.

Nutrition

   Calcium with vitamin D
   Vitamin C

Genitourinary/renal

   Torsemide
   Saw palmetto (What does evidence reveal about the use of this supplement?)
   Be aware of aspirin's alterations to this system.

Musculoskeletal

Cyclobenzaprine
Calcium with vitamin D

Endocrine

None specific

Integumentary

None specific

Immune

Some of you will place vitamin C here; however, what does the research/evidence tell us about vitamin C?

Pain/comfort

Some may place cyclobenzaprine here. Also, some may place aspirin here; review why it is given to this individual.

After your assessment, you call the primary care provider and discuss your findings. She requests that you send the patient to the emergency department. HHNS has developed related to his infection.

The treatment of his HHNS will center on reversing the dehydration, hyperglycemia, and electrolyte imbalances. Rehydration is the priority here. The type of solution determines cellular integrity. With the addition of insulin (to decrease the glucose) to the infusion, potassium must be monitored because of insulin's similar effect on potassium. Magnesium and potassium levels need to be monitored together because magnesium affects potassium and visa versa. The glucose levels are monitored to prevent hypoglycemia; when glucose reaches a certain level, dextrose is then added to stabilize glucose levels and prevent them from falling to dangerous levels.

Physician Orders

☑ Self-Query: Possible Answers

The patient now has two new medications and has been diagnosed with type II diabetes mellitus (DM).

Rosiglitazone (Avandia) 4 mg orally daily: rosiglitazone is used in type II DM. Medication increases muscle sensitivity to insulin in muscle and inhibits the liver from producing glucose (gluconeogenesis).

Metformin (Glucophage) 500 mg orally twice daily: metformin is also used in type II DM. Metformin decreases liver glucose production, decreases glucose absorption in the gastrointestinal tract, and works to promote cellular uptake of glucose. Rosiglitazone can be used alone or with diet and exercise to improve glycemic index. Rosiglitazone is usually combined with Metformin.

Case Study Inquiry
43

Vocabulary

Self-Query

Before attempting to work the case study, define each of the vocabulary words. Although the words may have several subheadings, it will give you a place to begin your inquiry.

Antipsychotic medications

_____

Dystonia

_____

Extrapyramidal symptoms

_____

Hallucination

_____

Lithium

_____

Psychosis

_____

Your new patient is a 30-year-old white female admitted from the emergency department. She is unkempt in appearance. She approached a couple on the street and became extremely agitated when they tried to walk away from her. They called the police. The police brought her to the hospital after noticing that she had several bruises and cuts. Presently, she is extremely paranoid and agitated.

Home Medications

Medication reconciliation upon this admission: Unable to determine

Allergies

Unable to determine

Physician Orders I

2 mg lorazepam (Ativan) IM
100 mg diphenhydramine (Benadryl) IM
10 mg haloperidol (Haldol) IM

Using a drug book or pharmacology text that contains the mechanism of action, unlabeled uses, and pharmacokinetics for medications, answer the following questions. Make answers specific to this scenario.

Before searching for the medications in a drug text, what do I know about these medications? Do I know the recommended dose of, the recommended route for, and the best time of day to give these medications? Do I know what lab results I need regarding each medication? Do I know the approved use of each medication? What is a possible medical diagnosis in the case related to each medication?

Lorazepam

_____

_____

Diphenhydramine

_____

_____

Haloperidol

_____

_____

Nursing Process

Self-Query

What nursing assessment will I perform regarding each medication? What planning and implementation do I need to do for each medication? How do I evaluate each medication's effectiveness?

Lorazepam

_____

_____

Diphenhydramine

_____

_____

Haloperidol

_____

_____

What classification is lorazepam? Why is it usually given? Do I know why the physician ordered it for this individual?

_____

_____

What classification is diphenhydramine? Why is it usually given? How is it given? Do I know why the physician ordered diphenhydramine for this individual?

_____

_____

Physician Orders II

The physician prescribes the following:

Admit for psychiatric evaluation

Chlorpromazine (Thorazine) 200 mg orally twice a day

Self-Query

What classification is chlorpromazine? Why is it usually given? List three different reasons for giving chlorpromazine. How is it given? Do I know why the physician ordered chlorpromazine for this individual?

_____

_____

The patient is now more controlled and refuses the medication, stating, "That drug makes my muscles jerk and I walk funny. I do not want to take it."

With which symptoms is the patient concerned? How does chlorpromazine cause these symptoms?

_____

_____

The physician changes the medication to:

Ziprasidone (Geodon) 80 mg orally twice a day

The patient says she will try the medication and will keep taking it if it does not have the effects that the other medication has on her.

What classification is ziprasidone? Why is it usually given? How is it given? Do I know why the physician ordered ziprasidone for this individual?

_____

_____

In further discussion, the patient reveals that she stopped taking her medications because she could not deal with the side effects. She has decided that the ziprasidone will work. After 3 days in the hospital, the patient recovers and is being discharged.

What teaching should be done so that this scenario does not happen again?

_____

_____

43

Because you can find answers to the self-queries in numerous texts, you will not find the answers to all of them here. However, you will find discussion of the individual case. The scenario relates to medications used in the dual diagnosis of mental illness and substance abuse; therefore, purposefully look into the medication use and vocabulary as they relate to these factors.

Vocabulary

When reviewing the vocabulary words, you might want to ask several questions: who, what, where, when, why, and how. This should give you a much broader understanding of each word.

Do yourself a favor and do not just give the shortest and simplest answer. Use the following example of hallucination: Instead of answering, "A hallucination is hearing, seeing, feeling, smelling, and even tasting things that are not real," ask:

Who is at risk for **hallucination**? How do medications treat hallucinations?

☑ Self-Query: Possible Answers

When defining the remainder of the vocabulary words, ask the following questions:

What is the mechanism of action in **antipsychotic medications**? What are the main side effects of these medications?

What is **dystonia**? Who is at risk?

What are **extrapyramidal symptoms (EPSs)**? How are they caused by antipsychotic medications?

Is **lithium** a drug used to treat hallucinations? Why is lithium used?

What is a **psychosis**?

Physician Orders I

☑ Self-Query: Possible Answers

The individual is experiencing a psychotic episode and needs emergency treatment before she harms herself or the emergency department staff.

2 mg lorazepam (Ativan) IM: lorazepam is a benzodiazepine. Its principal use is for anxiety. The patient is receiving it because it is fast acting and is useful against panic anxiety. In severely agitated individuals, it is administered in conjunction with haloperidol.

100 mg dipenhydramine (Benadryl) IM: diphenhydramine is a first-generation antihistamine and has anticholinergic effects. In addition, its mechanism of action on H_1 receptor sites causes sedation. Diphenhydramine is given both as a sedative and to counteract possible EPS side effects of the haloperidol.

10 mg haloperidol (Haldol) IM: haloperidol is an antipsychotic medication. It is considered a butyrophenone. Haloperidol blocks dopamine receptors and is effective against delusions and hallucinations. It causes EPS, particularly dystonia, in older patients. Haloperidol and dipenhydramine are not

usually combined in a syringe; however, some healthcare professionals give it in one injection. Some nurses place haloperidol in one syringe and lorazepam/dipenhydramine in another.

Chlorpromazine (Thorazine) 200 mg orally twice a day: chlorpromazine is an antipsychotic medication. It blocks dopamine receptors, which leads to its effects on the EPS. It also blocks serotonin receptors, histamine receptors, and adrenergic receptors. It has anticholinergic side effects because it blocks acetylcholine receptors. It effectively treats schizophrenia, manic episodes in bipolar disorder, and hiccups.

Physician Orders II

☑ Self-Query: Possible Answers

Ziprasidone (Geodon): ziprasidone is an antipsychotic medication with actions similar to chlorpromazine. It blocks, to some extent, receptors of dopamine, serotonin, acetylcholine, and histamine H_1. Ziprasidone is given only after an ECG has been evaluated because of its ability to prolong the QT/QTc interval.

See if the patient will attend a support group. The nurse should give the patient and family materials to contact a local chapter of the National Alliance for the Mentally Ill (NAMI). Stress to the patient that she needs to keep taking the medicine. If the side effects are unbearable, she needs to come back. Contact a psychiatric crisis center before the patient leaves and have a staff member talk with her.

Case Study Inquiry

44

Vocabulary

⸮ Self-Query

Before attempting to work the case study, define the vocabulary words. Although the words may have several subheadings, it will give you a place to begin your inquiry.

Acid-fast bacilli
_____

Fungal infections
_____

Lymphadenopathy
_____

Multidrug resistance
_____

Mycobacterium
_____

Night sweats
_____

Opportunistic infections
_____

Pneumonia
_____

Protozoa infections
_____

Tuberculosis (TB)
_____

Your new patient is a 45-year-old white female admitted from the emergency department. She is placed on droplet precautions because of a productive cough and fever of unknown origin (FUO, 101.3°F). She is unkempt in appearance and smells as if she has not bathed in quite some time. It is not possible to assess recent weight loss; however, she weighs 110 pounds and is 5′6″ tall. She attempted to sleep at a women's shelter this evening, where a worker noticed that she was extremely short of breath. During the night, the worker reported that the woman was coughing all night and coughed what looked like bloody sputum into a handkerchief. The worker brought her to the hospital immediately.

Home Medications

Medication reconciliation upon this admission:
The patient says that she does not receive any medications on a regular basis and that she does not have any allergies.

Physician Orders I

IV normal saline @ 125 mL/hr

PPD skin test

Sputum smear and culture

Complete blood count

Sedimentation rate

Liver function panel

BUN and creatinine

Nutritional consult

Self-Query

Why is the PPD test administered? What does PPD mean? How is it administered? What part of the body is tested? How will you explain the procedure? How will you know if it is negative? How will you know if it is positive? What body systems will you assess? What will the treatment be if it is positive?

_____

_____

Could the physician have used a QFT-G test in place of the PPD? If QFT-G test was obtained, how would it have been different from the PPD test?

_____

Why is the sputum smear and culture obtained? What is being assessed? How is a sputum smear and culture obtained? How will you know if it is negative? How will you know if it is positive? What body systems will you assess? What will the treatment be if it is positive?

_____

_____

_____

Physician Orders II

The physician prescribes the following:

Isoniazid 300 mg orally daily

Pyridoxine HCL 100 mg orally daily

Rifampin 600 mg orally daily

Pyrazinamide 500 mg orally daily

Ethambutol 500 mg orally daily

Self-Query

What classification is isoniazid?

_____

What classification is pyridoxine? What is another name for pyridoxine? What symptoms arise when a person has a pyridoxine deficiency? Why does pyridoxine need to be given with isoniazid?

_____

_____

What classification are these medications? What lab results are to be monitored? What major side effects are to be considered?

Rifampin

_____

_____

Pyrazinamide

_____

_____

Ethambutol

_____

_____

The patient begins to feel better and asks why she is taking four drugs for her lung disease. She has also been informed that she will take all these medications for 2 months. Then, for another 4 months, she will take the following medications:

Isoniazid 300 mg orally daily

Pyridoxine HCL 100 mg orally daily

Rifampin 600 mg orally daily

She asks you to explain the reasons for this schedule. She also wants you to tell her why she must visit an eye doctor and have monthly blood drawn to check her liver. A social worker has discovered that she has a son who is willing to care for her and ensure that she receives her medications.

Develop two nursing diagnoses for this patient (NANDA) in regard to the medications.

_____

_____

Develop at least three patient outcomes (NOC) in regard to the medications.

_____

_____

_____

Develop at least three patient interventions (NIC) in regard to the medications.

_____

_____

_____

Synopsis

44

Because you can find answers to the self-queries in numerous texts, you will not find the answers to all of them here. However, you will find discussion of the individual case. The scenario relates to medications used to treat pulmonary disease; therefore, purposefully look into medication use and vocabulary as they relate to these factors.

Vocabulary

When reviewing the vocabulary words, you might want to ask several questions: who, what, where, when, why, and how. This should give you a much broader understanding of each word.

Do yourself a favor and do not just give the shortest and simplest answer. Use the following example of opportunistic infection: Instead of answering, "Opportunistic infection is when a pathogen infects a person's body," ask:

What is an **opportunistic infection**? Who is at risk?

☑ Self-Query: Possible Answers

When defining the remainder of the vocabulary words, ask the following questions:

What does it mean to be acid-fast? What is **acid-fast bacilli**?

What is a **fungal infection**? How is it treated?

How is **lymphadenopathy** diagnosed? Who is at risk?

What causes **multidrug-resistant** bacteria? How can that be avoided?

What disease is caused by *Mycobacterium*? How is it treated?

What diseases are known for **night sweats**?

What is a **protozoa infection**? How is treated?

How does a person acquire **pneumonia**? How is it treated?

How does a person acquire **tuberculosis (TB)**? Why is TB treated with at least two medications?

Physician Orders I

☑ Self-Query: Possible Answers

The PPD was used to determine whether the individual had developed an immune response to the bacterium that causes TB. The response occurs if someone currently has TB, was exposed to it in the past, or has received the BCG vaccine against TB (which is not used in the United States). PPD stands for purified protein derivative.

A 0.1 mL of 5 tuberculin units is injected intradermally (just below the skin) of the forearm. A tuberculin syringe using a ¼- to ½-inch, 27-gauge needle is used. If the intradermal injection is done correctly, an elevation of the skin (a wheal) 6–10 mm in diameter is produced. It is quickly absorbed by the body.

The person reading the site looks for an induration. The patient's test was read at 48 and 72 hours after the injection. This person may or may not be immunocompromised. The reading will be different in otherwise healthy individuals. If her immune system is normal, induration greater than or equal to 15 mm is considered a positive skin test. If blisters appear, the test is considered positive. If she has kidney disease or diabetes, 10 mm of induration is considered a positive skin test result. If she is immunocompromised, 5 mm of induration is considered a positive skin test result. Induration of less than 2 mm without blistering is considered a negative skin test. Her test was 10 mm at 48 hours.

The QuantiFERON TB Gold test (QFT-G) is another way to detect the presence of TB in an individual and can be used in all cases in which the PPD is currently used.

An acid-fast culture refers to the process of detection, growth, isolation, identification, and antibiotic susceptibility testing of the bacteria that cause pulmonary TB. Remember that this individual is homeless, is most likely malnourished, and has active TB.

Physician Orders II

☑ Self-Query: Possible Answers

The physician prescribes:

Isoniazid 300 mg orally daily: isoniazid (INH) is used to treat TB or prevent its return (reactivation). INH is never used alone to treat active TB because resistance to INH by the bacterium develops quickly. INH also has the ability to inhibit the MAO enzyme, so this must be considered when dosing to depressed individuals. Liver enzymes are monitored. Peripheral neuropathy is a major side effect. INH destroys the cellular wall of bacteria.

Pyridoxine HCL 100 mg orally daily: in this individual, pyridoxine (vitamin B6) is used to prevent vitamin B6 deficiency. INH inhibits the metabolism of vitamin B6, which will lead to peripheral neuropathy. Because the patient is most likely undernourished, she is at high risk for peripheral neuropathy.

Rifampin 600 mg orally daily: rifampin is an antibiotic and is not used alone because of the ability of TB to develop resistance. It also inhibits cell wall reconstruction. Liver enzymes are monitored. Also assess for pancreatitis. Instruct the patient that body fluids will turn a red-orange color and that this is harmless, and that alternative birth control methods other than the pill should be used, if this is a possibility.

Pyrazinamide 500 mg orally daily: pyrazinamide is an antituberculosis agent. It can be bacteriostatic or bactericidal depending on the concentration of the drug at the site of infection. Liver enzymes are monitored.

Ethambutol 500 mg orally daily: ethambutol (EMB) is a bacteriostatic medication used against *Mycobacterium tuberculosis*. It is given in combination with INH, rifampin, and pyrazinamide. Liver enzymes are monitored. An eye exam is also needed. It is known to cause optic neuropathy and peripheral neuritis as well as liver dysfunction.

Regarding the patient's active TB, INH, rifampin, and pyrazinamide will be continued for the entire first 2 months. Ethambutol may be discontinued after the drug sputum cultures show that her bacterium is susceptible to both INH and rifampin. Because she was homeless, malnourished, and symptomatic of and positive for TB (skin and sputum cultures), she received a thorough physical examination. This included a chest x-ray, bacteriologic studies, and serology for HIV. She tested negative for HIV. She went to live with her son.

Case Study Inquiry

45

Vocabulary

☞ Self-Query

Before attempting to work the case study, define each of the vocabulary words. Although the words may have several subheadings, it will give you a place to begin your inquiry.

Atrial kick

_____

B-type natriuretic peptide (BNP)

_____

Blood urea nitrogen (BUN)

_____

Creatinine

_____

Ejection fraction

_____

Nebulizer

_____

Recent History

You are completing a full assessment on a 68-year-old female patient admitted to your intensive care unit from the emergency department. She has a left femoral head fracture from a fall. She developed respiratory depression after receiving a 4-mg morphine IV push. She then received naloxone (Narcan) 0.2 mg IV. Admitting vital signs: blood pressure 90/50; heart rate 118; respiratory rate 8.

☞ Self-Query

What classification is each of the prescribed medications? Why would the patient have received each medication? What geriatric concerns should have been addressed? What major side effects should have been considered?

Morphine

_____

_____

Naloxone

_____

_____

What is the explanation of the vital signs in regard to the morphine?

_____

How should naloxone affect the respiratory rate? How should naloxone affect the pain level?

_____

_____

Home Medications

You are conducting the medication reconciliation for this patient. She has the following medications and instructions in her purse.

Aspirin (ASA) 81 mg 1 tab orally chewed daily

Candesartan (Atacand) 16 mg orally daily

Furosemide (Lasix) 20 mg orally twice daily (9 a.m. and 1 p.m.)

Ibuprofen 200 mg 1–2 tabs daily for pain

Magnesium hydroxide (Milk of Magnesia) 30 mL daily

Self-Query

Using a drug book or pharmacology text that contains the mechanism of action, unlabeled uses, and pharmacokinetics for medications, answer the following questions. Make answers specific to this scenario.

What do I know about these medications? Do I know the recommended dose of, the recommended route for, and the best time of day to give these medications? Do I know what lab results I need regarding each medication? Do I know the approved use of each medication? Do I know the most common diseases treated by the listed medications? Are any off-label uses approved for each drug?

Aspirin

_____

_____

Candesartan

_____

_____

Furosemide

_____

_____

Ibuprofen

_____

_____

Magnesium hydroxide

_____

_____

What has research revealed about combining ibuprofen with aspirin when aspirin is prescribed for cardiac use?

_____

Do I know the individual's past medical history by looking at the medication list?

_____

_____

Body Systems

Self-Query

Be prepared to defend your answers.

Can I place each medication under the body system that it commonly affects?

Neurological

_____

Cardiovascular

_____

Hematological

_____

Pulmonary

_____

Gastrointestinal

_____

Nutrition

_____

Genitourinary/renal

_____

Musculoskeletal

_____

Endocrine

_____

Integumentary

_____

Immune

_____

Pain/comfort

_____

Nursing Process

Self-Query

The patient knows that she has to have hip repair surgery and fears that she is now allergic to morphine.

What instructions can you give the patient about pain management that will assure her that she will be able to take morphine after surgery?

_____

_____

She wants to know if meperidine (Demerol) would be a better choice. How will you answer this question? Explain your answer.

_____

_____

Synopsis

45

Because you can find answers to the self-queries in numerous texts, you will not find the answers to all of them here. However, you will find discussion of the individual case. The scenario relates to medications used in pain relief; therefore, purposefully look into the medication use and vocabulary as they relate to these factors.

Vocabulary

When reviewing the vocabulary words, you might want to ask several questions: who, what, where, when, why, and how. This should give you a much broader understanding of each word.

Do yourself a favor and do not just give the shortest and simplest answer. Use the following example of BUN: Instead of answering, "BUN is blood urea nitrogen," ask:

What does the **BUN** measure? How is it altered by age?

☑ Self-Query: Possible Answers

When defining the remainder of the vocabulary words, ask the following questions:

What is **atrial kick**? What percentage does it contribute to ventricular volume? What happens when it is not present?

What does the **BNP** measure? What does it mean when BNP is elevated? Give more than one reason.

What does the **creatinine** measure? How is it altered by age?

What is an **ejection fraction**? What does it reveal to us? What is a normal ejection fraction?

How is a **nebulizer** used? Why is a nebulizer used?

Recent History

☑ Self-Query: Possible Answers

The patient received morphine, an opioid analgesic, for severe pain related to her fall and hip pain. In therapeutic doses, there should be very little alteration of the cardiovascular system. However, she has received a dose that obviously caused respiratory depression, one of the most serious adverse effects. The hypotension is likely related to the alteration of the baroreceptor reflex. In addition, the vasodilation of arterioles and veins from morphine induced histamine release. Also, she could have undetected blood loss. However, find out her normal blood pressure before becoming concerned with something other than her respirations. Geriatric individuals are very sensitive to the respiratory effects of morphine.

Naloxone (Narcan) is an opioid antagonist and is used as an antidote when an individual receives too much of an opioid. When this medication was administered to reverse respiratory depression, it also negated the pain-relieving effect of the morphine. Remember this in the future if you administer naloxone to reverse postoperative opioid depression; the dose must be carefully administered to avoid reversing postoperative pain control.

Home Medications

✓ **Self-Query: Possible Answers**

Aspirin (ASA) 81 mg 1 tab orally chewed daily: used here as an antiplatelet

Candesartan (Atacand) 16 mg orally daily: angiotensin II receptor antagonist (hypertension)

Furosemide (Lasix) 20 mg orally twice daily (9 a.m. and 1 p.m.): high-loop diuretic (edema)

Ibuprofen 200 mg 1–2 tabs daily for pain: nonsteroidal anti-inflammatory

Magnesium hydroxide (Milk of Magnesia) 30 mL daily: self-medicates over-the-counter for constipation

Aspirin and ibuprofen together may increase the risk for gastrointestinal bleeding. The combination of aspirin (used as an antiplatelet medication) and other NSAIDs such as ibuprofen (used for pain) may lead to a drug-to-drug interaction that reduces aspirin's antiplatelet action.

Body Systems

✓ **Self-Query: Possible Answers**

Neurological

> None specific

Cardiovascular

> Aspirin
> Furosemide
> Candesartan

Hematological

> Aspirin

Pulmonary

> None specific

Gastrointestinal

> Magnesium hydroxide
> Also be aware of how aspirin and ibuprofen alter this system.

Nutrition

> None specific

Genitourinary/renal

> Furosemide
> Also be aware of how aspirin and ibuprofen alter this system

Musculoskeletal

> Ibuprofen

Endocrine

> None specific

Integumentary

> None specific

Immune

   None specific

Pain/comfort

   Ibuprofen

Some may place aspirin here, which in this case is not incorrect; however, see the dosage and why it is given. Her low-dose (81 mg) aspirin is used for myocardial infarction (MI) or stroke prevention. Higher doses increase the risk of bleeding but do not provide additional protection against stroke or MI.

She is not allergic to morphine, and the dose is adjusted to her system. Explain to her what happened.

Demerol is not a better choice. Meperidine (Demerol) is an opioid analgesic. It has many of the same side effects as morphine. In addition, it can only be used for a few days before a toxic metabolite called normeperidine accumulates and causes seizures in some individuals. She will receive pain medication before surgery. After surgery and upon discharge, she will be placed on an oral pain reliever and possible muscle relaxer.

Case Study Inquiry

46

Vocabulary

♟ Self-Query

Before attempting to work the case study, define each of the vocabulary words. Although the words may have several subheadings, it will give you a place to begin your inquiry.

Convulsions

_____

Depression

_____

Epilepsy

_____

Generalized seizures

_____

Gingival hyperplasia

_____

Hirsutism

_____

Partial seizures

_____

The daughter of a 53-year-old female patient has driven her to the emergency room after witnessing a series of jerking motions and loss of consciousness. The daughter has brought a list of the patient's medications to the hospital.

Home Medications

Acetaminophen (Tylenol) ES 1–2 capsules orally daily as needed

Bisacodyl 10-mg suppositories once daily for constipation

Calcium supplementation of at least 1200 mg per day

Docusate 100 mg orally daily

Ibandronate (Boniva) 150 mg orally once a month

Phenobarbital 250 mg orally daily

Phenytoin 400 mg orally daily

Sertraline 50 mg orally twice a day

Vitamin D 400 IU orally daily

Using a drug book or pharmacology text that contains the mechanism of action, unlabeled uses, and pharmacokinetics for medications, answer the following questions. Make answers specific to this scenario.

Match the medications to the appropriate medical diagnosis history.

Acetaminophen

_____

Bisacodyl

_____

Calcium supplementation

_____

Docusate

_____

Ibandronate

_____

Phenobarbital

_____

Phenytoin

_____

Sertraline

_____

Vitamin D

_____

Do I know the individual's past medical history by looking at the medication list?

_____

_____

Body Systems

? **Self-Query**

Be prepared to defend your answers.

Can I place each medication under the body system that it commonly affects?

Neurological

_____

Cardiovascular

_____

Hematological

_____

Pulmonary

_____

Gastrointestinal

_____

Nutrition

_____

Genitourinary/renal

Musculoskeletal

Endocrine

Integumentary

Immune

Pain/comfort

Synopsis

46

Because you can find answers to the self-queries in numerous texts, you will not find the answers to all of them here. However, you will find discussion of the individual case. The scenario relates to medications used in neurological diseases. Therefore, purposefully look into the medication use and vocabulary as they relate to these factors.

Vocabulary

When reviewing the vocabulary words, you might want to ask several questions: who, what, where, when, why, and how. This should give you a much broader understanding of each word.

Do yourself a favor and do not just give the shortest and simplest answer. Use the following example of convulsions: Instead of answering, "Convulsions are a type of seizure," ask:

Who is at risk for **convulsions**? What medications might cause a seizure (legal and illegal)? Can the words *convulsion* and *seizure* be interchangeable?

☑ Self-Query: Possible Answers

When defining the remainder of the vocabulary words, ask the following questions:

What causes **depression**? Why is it common in seizure disorders?

What is **epilepsy**? How is it diagnosed?

What are **generalized seizures**? How are they categorized? How are they treated?

What is **gingival hyperplasia**? Which medication is known to cause this?

What is **hirsutism**? How is it treated?

What is a **partial seizure**? How are they categorized? How are they treated?

Home Medications

☑ Self-Query: Possible Answers

Acetaminophen (Tylenol) ES 1–2 capsules orally daily as needed: acetaminophen is used to reduce pain and fever. Because of its common use and popularity, it can cause liver failure. It does not have an effect on inflammation.

Bisacodyl 10-mg suppositories once daily for constipation: bisacodyl directly stimulates the bowel muscles.

Calcium supplementation of at least 1200 mg per day: used to replace calcium. Calcium is recommended for healthy bones and is given in conjunction with the ibandronate. Calcium is used by the body for numerous functions: maintenance of bones and teeth, regulating heart rhythm, promoting normal blood clotting, promoting proper nerve and muscle function, and lowering blood pressure, just to name a few.

Docusate 100 mg orally daily: used in constipation. Docusate is a surfactant that is used as a stool softener.

Ibandronate (Boniva) 150 mg orally once a month: ibandronate is a biphosphate used in the treatment of postmenopausal osteoporosis. Individuals will require a routine bone mineral density (BMD) exam. The individual must be able to sit or stand at least 60 minutes after ingestion to allow the medication to absorb. Lying down can promote the development of esophagitis. This drug is not to be taken with any other medications and should be taken with a full glass of water.

Phenobarbital 250 mg orally daily: phenobarbital is a barbiturate and is used in the treatment of seizures. It promotes sensory cortex depression, decreases motor activity, and alters cerebellar function. All of this promotes drowsiness, sedation, and hypnosis. It is given here for seizure activity. This medication should be taken at bedtime.

Phenytoin (Dilantin) 400 mg orally daily: phenytoin is an anticonvulsant used in the treatment of grand mal-type seizures. The primary site of action appears to be the motor cortex. In the past, it has also been used as a cardiac medication. Hypotension usually occurs when the drug is administered rapidly by the intravenous route. Phenytoin is sometimes given IV for status epilepticus. It is also noted for coarsening of the facial features, enlargement of the lips, and gingival hyperplasia.

Sertraline 50 mg orally twice a day: sertraline, also known as Zoloft, is an antidepressant. It is classified as a selective serotonin reuptake inhibitor. It is given to this person to treat a panic disorder.

Vitamin D 400 IU orally daily: used to promote calcium absorption in the small intestine. Vitamin D is a fat-soluble vitamin. It is present in certain foods, is added to certain foods, and is available as a dietary supplement. It is produced internally when ultraviolet rays from sunlight strike the skin and trigger vitamin D synthesis. Here it is administered with the calcium to promote the absorption of calcium.

Body Systems

☑ Self-Query

Neurological

> Acetaminophen
> Sertraline
> Phenytoin
> Phenobarbital

Cardiovascular

> None specific

Hematological

> Ibandronate
> Calcium supplementation
> Vitamin D

Pulmonary

> None specific

Gastrointestinal

> Docusate
> Bisacodyl

Nutrition

> None specific; however, be aware that chronic use of docusate orally and in suppository form may alter the individual's nutritional status.

Genitourinary/renal

 None specific

Musculoskeletal

 Ibandronate
 Calcium supplementation
 Vitamin D
 Acetaminophen

Endocrine

 None specific

Integumentary

 None specific

Immune

 None specific

Pain/comfort

 Acetaminophen

Case Study Inquiry

47

Patient #1

A neurological patient is on your unit. You are reviewing the medications of a 33-year-old female admitted for surgery.

Home Medications

Aspirin (Ecotrin) 325 mg orally as needed for pain and fever

Dihydroergotamine (D.H.E. 45) intramuscularly 1-mg injection at onset of symptoms

Metoclopramide (Reglan) 20 mg orally at onset of symptoms

Propranolol (Inderal) LA 80 mg orally daily

Riboflavin (Vitamin B2) 400 mg orally daily

Topiramate (Topamax) 50 mg orally twice a day

Ubiquinone (Coenzyme Q10) 100 mg orally 3 times a day

Self-Query

What are these medications?

Aspirin

_____

Dihydroergotamine

_____

Metoclopramide

_____

Propranolol

_____

Riboflavin

_____

Topiramate

_____

Ubiquinone

_____

What could be the individual's primary diagnosis?

_____

Allergies

Feverfew

Self-Query

What is Feverfew? What is this substance and is it a prescription medication?

_____

Patient #2

A neurological patient is on your unit. History of present illness: You are reviewing the medications of an individual who reports, "My disease appears to be getting worse. I am here to see what can be done."

Home Medications

Aspirin (Ecotrin) 325 mg orally as needed for pain and fever

Prednisone 20 mg orally daily

Pyridostigmine 60 mg orally twice a day as maintenance dose

Physician Orders

Begin to taper prednisone

Begin azathioprine (Imuran) 50 mg orally daily

Self-Query

What are these medications?

Aspirin

_____

Prednisone

_____

Pyridostigmine

_____

Azathioprine

_____

What could be the individual's primary diagnosis?

_____

If there is a taper order, how long was the patient taking the prednisone? Write a plan to taper the prednisone.

_____

_____

Synopsis

47

Patient #1

The patient is experiencing migraine headaches.

Home Medications

☑ Self-Query: Possible Answers

Aspirin (Ecotrin) 325 mg orally as needed for pain and fever: Ecotrin is enteric-coated aspirin. Aspirin is salicylic acid and is used as an anti-inflammatory, antipyretic, and antithrombotic. The anti-inflammatory and analgesic effects of aspirin are roughly equivalent to those of other NSAIDs. Aspirin is used for its anti-inflammatory effect in treating migraines.

Dihydroergotamine (D.H.E. 45) 1 mg intramuscularly at onset of symptoms: dihydroergotamine binds to serotonin and dopamine receptors. It is given for migraines and is believed to act on intracranial vascular causing vasoconstriction. This leads to migraine relief when the migraine is caused by vasoconstriction of the vessels. This medication is prescribed when less vasoconstrictive medications are not effective.

Metoclopramide (Reglan) 20 mg orally at onset of symptoms: metoclopramide promotes tissue sensitivity to the neurotransmitter acetylcholine and promotes gastric motility. The nausea in migraines might be attributed to gastric stasis, a delayed emptying of the stomach; in these cases, a prokinetic medication such as metoclopramide alleviates the nausea.

Propranolol (Inderal) LA 80 mg orally daily: beta blockers are a class of drugs that block the effects of beta-adrenergic substances such as adrenaline (epinephrine). It is administered as a prophylaxis against migraines.

Riboflavin (Vitamin B_2) 400 mg orally daily: like all B vitamins, it is soluble in water. It plays a major role in the conversion of carbohydrates into sugar. The eight B vitamins, which are also known as vitamin B complex, are necessary to metabolize fat and proteins.

Topiramate (Topamax) 50 mg twice a day: anticonvulsant medication. Promotes the activity of GABA, a neurotransmitter; given as migraine prophylaxis.

Ubiquinone (Coenzyme Q10 [CoQ10]) 100 mg orally 3 times a day: ubiquinone is a fat-soluble, vitamin-like substance. It is produced by the human body and is necessary for the basic functioning of cells. CoQ10 levels are reported to decrease with age and to be decreased in some individuals. It is considered to have antioxidant properties. It decreases the severity of the patient's headaches.

Allergies

☑ Self-Query: Possible Answers

Feverfew: Feverfew is an herb that is thought to help prevent migraines, but research has not proved any benefit. The patient tried Feverfew and reported a red raised rash and increased nausea that lasted 24 hours.

Patient #2

The patient has myasthenia gravis.

Physician Orders

☑ Self-Query: Possible Answers

Aspirin (Ecotrin) 325 mg orally as needed for pain and fever: Ecotrin is enteric-coated aspirin. Aspirin is salicylic acid and is used as an anti-inflammatory, antipyretic, and antithrombotic. The anti-inflammatory and analgesic effects of aspirin are roughly equivalent to those of other NSAIDs. Because of its antithrombotic effects, aspirin is used to prevent or reduce the risk of myocardial infarction (MI) and transient ischemic attacks (TIAs).

Prednisone 20 mg orally daily: prednisone, a corticosteroid, decreases inflammation and is used in this case to reduce the number of antibodies produced (that is, for immunosuppression).

Pyridostigmine 60 mg orally twice a day as a maintenance dose: pyridostigmine is an anticholinesterase drug and promotes the body's use of acetylcholine (Ach). It blocks the enzyme that usually breaks down Ach. This allows the Ach to concentrate at the muscle receptor, which in turn allows a prolonged effect of the Ach from the nerves to the muscles.

To taper prednisone: 40 mg × 14 days, then 30 mg × 14 days, then 20 mg × 14 days, then 10 mg × 14 days, then 5 mg × 14 days.

Begin azathioprine (Imuran) 50 mg orally daily: azathioprine is also an immunosuppressant (see prednisone). However, it works differently than prednisone does. It is used in diseases in which activity of the immune system is important. It decreases the proliferation of T and B lymphocytes. It is thought that migraine in some cases may be an autoimmune reaction.

Case Study Inquiry

48

Case Presentation

You are the nurse working in an endocrinologist's office. The patient is a 40-year-old female who was diagnosed with an autoimmune disorder 10 years ago. She is a new referral from a rheumatologist.

She has developed severe headaches over the past month.

She experiences heart palpitations.

She also thinks she may be experiencing early menopause because of her "severe sweating."

Her blood glucose is high, as is her blood pressure.

Home Medications

Following are the patient's present medications:

Chloroquine (Plaquenil)

Folic acid 400 mcg every morning

Metformin (Glucophage) 850 mg once a day, taken with dinner at 5 p.m.

Naproxen 500 mg twice a day

Nebivolol (Bystolic) 5 mg orally daily

Paroxetine (Paxil) 20 mg at bedtime

Prednisone 20 mg orally every morning

Ranitidine (Zantac) 150 mg at bedtime

Vitamin B12 one tab daily

Self-Query

What are these medications? What can you explain about them?

Chloroquine

_____

Folic acid

_____

Metformin

_____

Naproxen

_____

Nebivolol

_____

Paroxetine

_____

Prednisone

_____

Ranitidine

_____

Vitamin B12

_____

Allergies

Methotrexate (MTX)

Azathioprine (Imuran)

? Self-Query

What are these medications? What can you explain about them?

Methotrexate

_____

Azathioprine

_____

Physician Orders

After a thorough evaluation, the patient is scheduled for an adrenalectomy.

? Self-Query

Why would she need an adrenalectomy?

_____

_____

What medications will be needed after a total adrenalectomy?

_____

_____

Synopsis

48

Case Presentation

Cushing's syndrome is caused by exposure to glucocorticoids, which are used to treat inflammatory diseases. The patient has taken prednisone and Solu-Medrol for psoriasis and rheumatoid disease over many years. This individual had adverse reactions to most of the newer anti-inflammatory medications for rheumatoid arthritis (RA). This is why she was on the continual dose of prednisone.

Home Medications

☑ Self-Query: Possible Answers

Chloroquine (Plaquenil): chloroquine is prescribed for the prevention and treatment of certain forms of malaria. However, in this case, it is used to treat the symptoms of RA such as swelling, inflammation, stiffness, and joint pain. How it works in RA is not really known.

Folic acid 400 mcg every morning: folic acid promotes the reproduction of new cells. This was added when she was prescribed the MTX, and it was not stopped.

Metformin (Glucophage) 850 mg once a day, taken with dinner at 5 p.m.: metformin is an antihyperglycemic medication. It provides increased glucose tolerance in individuals diagnosed with type II diabetes. Metformin decreases glucose production in the liver, decreases glucose absorption in the intestines, and improves glucose uptake and utilization in cells.

Naproxen 500 mg twice a day: naproxen is a nonsteroidal anti-inflammatory drug (NSAID) used here for RA pain.

Nebivolol (Bystolic) 5 mg orally daily: nebivolol provides relief from hypertension, possibly by decreasing heart rate and suppressing renin activity and decreasing peripheral vascular resistance.

Paroxetine (Paxil) 20 mg at bedtime: paroxetine is an antidepressant classified as a serotonin receptor reuptake inhibitor.

Prednisone 20 mg orally every morning: prednisone is an adrenocortical steroid (steroid produced in the adrenal glands). In this case, it is used as an anti-inflammatory for RA.

Ranitidine (Zantac) 150 mg at bedtime: ranitidine is a histamine-2 blocker. It decreases the acid produced in the stomach.

Vitamin B12 one tab daily: B12 promotes the reproduction of new cells, which is required for normal metabolism of carbohydrate, protein, and fat. It needs to be given because the folic acid may mask a B12 deficiency. B12 was added when the patient was prescribed the MTX and folate, and it was not stopped.

Allergies

☑ Self-Query: Possible Answers

Methotrexate (MTX): MTX is an antimetabolite and antifolate drug. It is used in cancer therapy and in treating autoimmune diseases such as RA. It acts by inhibiting the metabolism of folic acid.

Azathioprine (Imuran): azathioprine is used in diseases in which activity of the immune system is important. It decreases the proliferation of T and B lymphocytes.

Physician Orders

☑ Self-Query: Possible Answers

After a thorough evaluation, the patient is scheduled for an adrenalectomy. She has a pheochromocytoma, a tumor of the adrenal glands. These tumors secrete epinephrine, norepinephrine, and dopamine, which are known as catecholamines. Her prednisone dose may need to be increased.

Case Study Inquiry

49

Case Presentation

You are a nurse in a rehabilitation unit specializing in spinal cord injuries. The patient is moved to your unit after 2 months in the hospital recovering from a snowmobile accident. She hit a tree headfirst without her helmet. She is able to move her arms and has increased her upper body strength. However, she developed a stage 3 pressure ulcer on her coccyx area. She reports that the pain from the ulcer is increasing, and now, as she begins to be more mobile, she has an increasing burning sensation in her lower extremities.

Medications

Present pain medications:

Propoxyphene and acetaminophen (Darvocet-N) 100 mg orally every 6 hours as needed for pain

Referral: pain management specialist
Prescription for the following:

Propoxyphene and acetaminophen 100 mg orally every 8 hours

Fentanyl (Duragesic) patch 25 mcg/hour every 72 hours

Begin levetiracetam (Keppra) 500 mg orally at 9 p.m. × 2 days, then measure effects on leg pain; assess for other side effects and begin levetiracetam 500 mg orally 9 a.m. and 9 p.m.

What do you know about these medications?

Propoxyphene and acetaminophen

_____

_____

Fentanyl

_____

_____

Levetiracetam

_____

_____

What type of pain does this individual have?

_____

_____

Synopsis

49

Case Presentation

This individual presents with nociceptive- and neuropathic-type pains.

Medications

☑ **Self-Query: Possible Answers**

Nociceptive Pain

Darvocet-N 100 mg orally every 8 hrs (Note: it is no longer as needed): combination of 100 mg propoxyphene napsylate (an opioid analgesic) and 650 mg acetaminophen (nonopioid analgesic). The combination of propoxyphene and acetaminophen produces greater analgesia than that produced by either propoxyphene or acetaminophen administered alone. Propoxyphene napsylate is related to methadone.

Fentanyl (Duragesic) patch 25 mcg/hour every 72 hours: fentanyl is a transdermal patch. It is a schedule II opioid agonist and provides pain relief around the clock.

Neuropathic Pain

Levetiracetam (Keppra) 500 mg orally 9 a.m. and 9 p.m.: levetiracetam is an antiepileptic drug. It is thought that it reduces the nerve impulse conduction across synapses. This is the reason it can be used in neuropathic pain; it interrupts the nerve conduction that causes the pain.

Case Study Inquiry

50

Case Presentation

You are attempting to do medication reconciliation for a new patient. She has moved to the area and has set up an appointment to establish the physician you work with as her primary care provider. The clinic specializes in rheumatology and musculoskeletal disorders. She gives you the following list of medications; she says she has taken more medications than this in the past but has been maintained for a year with only the medications on this list.

Home Medications

Celecoxib (Celebrex) 100 mg orally daily

Cevimeline (Evoxac) 30 mg orally 3 times a day

Etanercept (Enbrel) subcutaneous injection 25-mg prefilled syringe

Losartan (Cozaar) 25 mg orally daily

Metaxalone (Skelaxin) 800 mg orally twice a day

Omeprazole (Prilosec) 40 mg orally daily

Tramadol 50 mg every 6 hours as needed

Ubiquinone (CoQ10) one capsule daily

Self-Query

What are these medications? Why are they given? What diseases are most likely treated with these medications?

Celecoxib

_____

_____

Cevimeline

_____

_____

Etanercept

_____

_____

Losartan

_____

_____

Metaxalone

_____

_____

Omeprazole

_____

_____

Tramadol

_____

_____

Ubiquinone

_____

_____

Synopsis

50

Case Presentation

The patient has lupus and Sjögren's syndrome.

Home Medications

☑ Self-Query: Possible Answers

Celecoxib (Celebrex) 100 mg orally daily: celecoxib is a nonsteroidal anti-inflammatory drug (NSAID). It is a COX-2 inhibitor.

Cevimeline (Evoxac) 30 mg orally 3 times a day: cevimeline is used to treat the symptom of dry mouth (xerostomia) in individuals with Sjögren's syndrome. It increases the activity of glands in the mouth and skin. It is a muscarinic agonist. It is a derivative of acetylcholine.

Etanercept (Enbrel) subcutaneous injection 25-mg prefilled syringe: etanercept is a medication used to treat autoimmune diseases. It interferes with and blocks tumor necrosis factor (TNF). TNF is a part of the immune system.

Losartan (Cozaar) 25 mg orally daily: losartan is an angiotensin II receptor, which is similar to an ACE inhibitor but without the detrimental side effects (cough, hyperkalemia). It works by blocking receptor sites from angiotensin II, therefore creating vasodilatation of arterioles and veins.

Metaxalone (Skelaxin) 800 mg orally twice a day: metaxalone is a muscle relaxant used to relax muscles and relieve pain. It may work by depressing the central nervous system.

Omeprazole (Prilosec) 40 mg orally daily: omeprazole is a proton pump inhibitor used to treat gastric acid disease.

Tramadol 50 mg every 6 hours as needed: tramadol is an analog of codeine and is used to relieve pain. It seems to work by blocking the uptake of norepinephrine and serotonin. It has low abuse potential.

Ubiquinone (Coenzyme Q10 [CoQ10]) 1 capsule daily: ubiquinone is a fat-soluble, vitamin-like substance. It is produced by the human body and is necessary for the basic functioning of cells. CoQ10 levels are reported to decrease with age and to be decreased in some individuals. It is considered to have antioxidant properties. It decreases the severity of the patient's headaches.

Index